Pocket Handbook of
Common Cardiac Arrhythmias: Recognition and Treatment

POCKET HANDBOOK OF
Common Cardiac Arrhythmias:
Recognition and Treatment

Anne E. Garrett, RN, BA, MA

Clinical Nurse III
Progressive Care Unit
Sibley Memorial Hospital
Washington, DC

Virginia Adams, RN

Staff Nurse
Progressive Care Unit
Sibley Memorial Hospital
Washington, DC

J.B. Lippincott Company
Philadelphia
London Mexico City New York St. Louis São Paulo Sydney

Sponsoring Editor: Paul Hill
Manuscript Editor: Rosanne Hallowell
Indexer: Deana Rees Fowler
Art Director: Tracy Baldwin
Design Coordinator: Earl Gerhart
Designer: Katharine Nichols
Production Supervisor: J. Corey Gray
Production Coordinator: Barney Fernandes
Compositor: Circle Graphics
Printer/Binder: R. R. Donnelley & Sons Company

6 5 4 3 2 1

Library of Congress Cataloging in Publication Data

Garrett, Anne E.
  Pocket handbook of common cardiac arrhythmias.

  Bibliography: p.
  Includes index.
  1. Arrhythmia—Handbooks, manuals, etc. I. Adams,
Virginia, 1947–   . II. Title. [DNLM: 1. Arrhythmia—
diagnosis—handbooks. 2. Arrhythmia—therapy—handbooks.
WG 39 G239p]
RC685.A65G34 1986   616.1′28   85-24
ISBN 0-397-54530-4

In fond memory of our fathers
and
loving honor of our mothers and brothers

Preface

Our idea for writing *Pocket Handbook of Common Cardiac Arrhythmias: Recognition and Treatment* arose from watching the perplexed expressions on colleagues' faces (and our own) as they scrambled through pages of numerous references on cardiac arrhythmias and their drug therapy. We needed something close at hand that would make such information readily available with special information on nursing implications. Frustration mounted . . . and then, "Why not write something to meet our needs?" Why not . . . .

This reference is designed as an on-the-spot resource to meet immediate needs. It is to be used to provide answers to problems as they arise on the job. No longer does one need to consult numerous references to gain knowledge about identifying arrhythmias, another for drug treatment and usual dosage, and still another to discover what the nurse should be alert for with patients having arrhythmias and receiving drug therapy. We attempted to delete extra verbiage and present material in a simple, straightforward manner.

This book may be used as a self-study primer to help the beginning student recognize common disorders of the cardiac rhythm, or it may be used as a beginning text in the classroom. Because of its simple format, it will be useful as a text for in-hospital training programs for nurses wishing to work in coronary care units. Programs for medical interns and residents may wish to use this book as a basic reference. Finally, it may serve as a basic reference for cardiac care units or as a personal reference for medical residents and cardiac care nurses.

Anatomy and electrophysiology are discussed only to the extent essential for interpretation of cardiac rhythms. From that point, the reader will be able to understand better the mechanisms and causes of arrhythmias.

It is our hope that this book will help make the complex work of the cardiac care nurse just a little simpler.

Anne E. Garrett, RN, BA, MA
Virginia Adams, RN

Acknowledgments

Appreciation especially goes to to our families for their moral support and faith in us. Also, special gratitude to Ellen B. Raffensperger, RN, CCRN, our colleague, who put us in touch with David T. Miller, Vice President at Lippincott, who encouraged us to pursue our dream, and to Paul R. Hill, Editor, who helped us realize our dream.

The content of this book has benefited significantly from reviews and invaluable suggestions by the following:

Phyllis Godwin Byles, RN, BSN
Former Head Nurse
Progressive Care Unit
Sibley Memorial Hospital
Washington, DC

Gary P. Fisher, MD, FACC
Chevy Chase, Maryland

Richard B. Glover, BS, CCPT
Cardiopulmonary Technologist
Sibley Memorial Hospital
Washington, DC

Janet Grinc, RN, BSN, CCRN
Head Nurse
Former Critical Care Instructor
Sibley Memorial Hospital
Washington, DC

Ken Ingignoli, RCPT
Cardiopulmonary Technologist
Sibley Memorial Hospital
Washington, DC

Lewis C. Lipson, MD, FACC
Chevy Chase, Maryland

Joan Vincent, RN, MSN
Clinical Instructor, Critical Care
Sibley Memorial Hospital
Washington, DC

A special "thank you" from Virginia Adams to her mentors, Sandy A. Fury, MD, and Phyllis Snyder, RN, and from Anne Garrett to Joann "Griff" Alspach, RN, MSN, CCRN; also, to our nursing instructors who made us what we are today—you know who you are.

Contents

And the Beat Goes On:

Cardiac Anatomy and

Physiology

The heart is the center of the cardiovascular system. Although its size varies with the size of the individual, it is roughly the equivalent of two clenched fists. In the fully developed adult, it weighs between 11 and 16 ounces. It lies in the chest cavity between the two lungs, with the right atrium and ventricle more toward the anterior than the left atrium and ventricle.

The heart is a hollow, muscular organ that has only one function: *to pump*. Oxygen-poor blood received from the body is pumped to the pulmonary system to pick up oxygen. This oxygenated blood then is pumped back to the heart and out to the body. The heart forces blood to flow by contractions called *systoles*. Each systole is followed by a period of rest, or *diastole*. The heart must be sensitive to ever-changing demands of the peripheral circulation including exercise, emotional excitement, digestion, temperature, and positional changes.

The heart is composed of four chambers: (1) the right atrium, (2) the right ventricle, (3) the left atrium and (4) the left ventricle. The right and left sides are divided by the septal wall. So that the blood will be pumped in the proper direction, the heart has valves to prevent backflow or regurgitation (Fig. 1). Thus, when the right ventricle contracts forcing blood through the pulmonary artery, the tricuspid valve prevents regurgitation into the right atrium, from whence it came. The blood that has just been pumped into the pulmonary artery cannot flow back into the right ventricle, which is in diastole, because the pulmonic valve is closed during the period of relaxation. A similar process is occurring at the same time on the left side of the heart. The mitral valve (bicuspid valve) prevents regurgitation from the left ventricle into the left atrium during systole, while the aortic valve prevents its return from the pulmonary vein into the left ventricle during diastole (Fig. 2).

The ability to contract is inherent in the heart wall (myocardium). If the ventricles were separated entirely from the

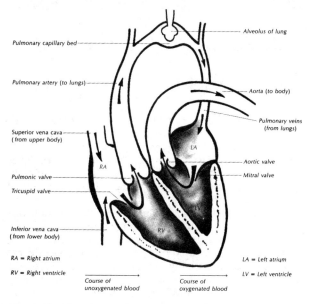

Pulmonary capillary bed

Pulmonary artery (to lungs)

Superior vena cava
(*from upper body*)

Pulmonic valve

Tricuspid valve

Inferior vena cava
(*from lower body*)

Alveolus of lung

Aorta (to body)

Pulmonary veins
(*from lungs*)

Aortic valve

Mitral valve

LA

RA

LV

RV

RA = Right atrium

RV = Right ventricle

LA = Left atrium

LV = Left ventricle

Course of
unoxygenated blood

Course of
oxygenated blood

Fig. 1. Anatomy of the heart.

remainder of the heart, under certain conditions they would continue to contract regularly at approximately 30 beats per minute. The atrial walls also can beat independently, at a faster rate than the ventricular walls.

The Heart's Conduction System

The natural pacemaker of the heart is the sinoatrial or S-A node. It is located in the posterior wall of the right atrium near the opening of the superior vena cava, where normally all the heart's beats originate. It is through the S-A node that certain autonomic nervous centers in the brain control the heartbeat's rate. Sympathetic nerve fibers speed it, vagus nerve fibers slow it. The balance of the sympathetic and vagus nerve systems controls the S-A node and thus determines the heartbeat's rate.

Hence, a single electrical impulse generated by and originating in the S-A node, the heart's pacemaker, normally causes every muscular contraction of the heart. The impulse travels by way of conduction pathways through the right and left atrial walls, exciting their immediate contraction. The impulse continues to travel to the fibers called the "bundle of His," or atrioventricular bundle. Shortly beyond the A-V node, the pathway divides into the right and left bundle branches. The Purkinje fibers, located at the end of each bundle branch, conduct the impulse from the A-V node to the right and left ventricles, distributing it throughout both ventricular walls stimulating them to contract and force blood out to the body.

Each normal heartbeat, therefore, is a precisely timed and executed sequence of events which can be described as follows:

1. Electrical discharge initiates in S-A node ⟶
2. Atria contract and empty into corresponding ventricles, which are, at the time, in diastole ⟶
3. Ventricles contract simultaneously after approximately a 0.10-second interval. The right ventricle ejects systemic venous blood into the pulmonary artery, then to the lungs to pick up oxygen. The left ventricle ejects oxygenated blood from the pulmonary system into the aorta and systemic circulation.

Electrocardiography

The electrical mechanism of depolarization and repolarization causes the heart's muscle cells to contract and relax as a unit. When at rest, the myocardial cells are polarized, that is, the number of positive ions outside each cell is equal to the number of negative ions inside each cell. At the beginning of each cardiac cycle, when the S-A node emits an electrical impulse, the polarized cells become depolarized or electrically imbalanced: the cell becomes positive on the inside and negative on the outside. This causes the cells to contract. When the electrical impulse passes through the cells, they become repolarized and are again in balance. The sum total of this process is the cardiac cycle.

Most electrical activity over the trunk of an inactive person emanates from the heart's depolarizing and repolarizing sequences. The electrocardiograph converts the electrical currents into mechanical energy and records them by means of stylus deflections produced by heat con-

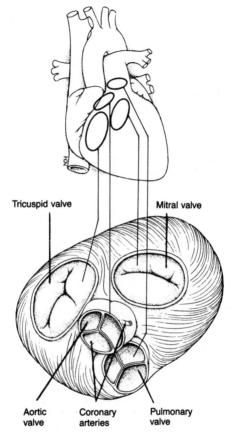

Tricuspid valve   Mitral valve

Aortic   Coronary   Pulmonary
valve   arteries   valve

Fig. 2. The heart's valves prevent backflow of blood.

tact on graphic paper. These recordings are called electro-cardiograms (ECGs). The paper moves at a constant rate so that electrical oscillations are recorded in relation to the duration over which it occurs. The composite of all heart cells' action potential at one particular time is represented by each deflection on the ECG.

Deflection is determined by the electrodes' position on the body. Thus, an upward deflection is positive and a

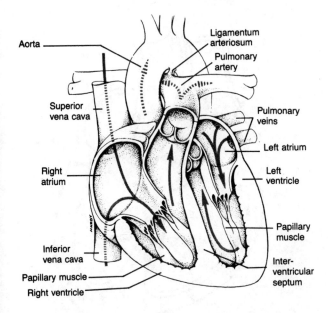

Aorta

Ligamentum arteriosum

Pulmonary artery

Superior vena cava

Pulmonary veins

Left atrium

Right atrium

Left ventricle

Papillary muscle

Inferior vena cava

Inter-ventricular septum

Papillary muscle

Right ventricle

downward deflection is negative. Amplitude is determined by the amount of electrical potential between electrodes at that specific instant. Much can be deduced about the heart's activity from the figures recorded on graphic paper.

Figures 3 and 4 depict components of the cardiac cycle as they relate to movement on the electrocardiograph.

ECG paper is gridded using standardized dimensions (Fig. 5). The light vertical and horizontal lines are exactly 1 mm apart. Every fifth line, both vertically and horizontally, is darker and heavier; these darker lines are 5 mm apart. The horizontal axis, read from left to right, represents time. At a standard recording speed of 25 mm/second, each 1-mm interval = 0.04 second. The vertical axis represents the amplitude of the ECG figures.

Three measurements are required for interpretation of cardiac rhythm: (1) PR interval, (2) width of QRS complex, and (3) rate, both atrial and ventricular.

The PR interval starts with the first deflection of atrial depolarization and ends with the first deflection of the QRS complex. It should measure no less than 0.12 second and no greater than 0.20 second.

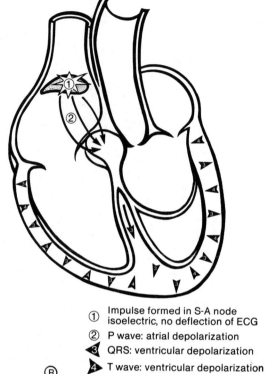

① Impulse formed in S-A node
   isoelectric, no deflection of ECG
② P wave: atrial depolarization
③ QRS: ventricular depolarization
④ T wave: ventricular depolarization

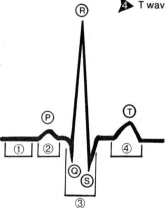

Fig. 3. The cardiac cycle and the ECG.

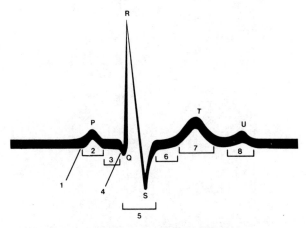

Fig. 4. Electrical events of the cardiac cycle.

Electrical Event	ECG Representation
1. Impulse from sinus node	Not visible
2. Depolarization of atria	P wave
3. Depolarization of A–V node	Isoelectric
4. Repolarization of atria	Obscured by QRS complex
5. Depolarization of ventricles	QRS complex
a. Intraventricular septum	a. Initial portion
b. Right & left ventricles	b. Central & terminal portions
6. Activated state of ventricles immediately after depolarization	ST segment: isoelectric
7. Repolarization of ventricles	T wave
8. After-potentials following repolarization of ventricles	U wave

The QRS complex starts with the first deflection from baseline caused by ventricular depolarization and ends with return to baseline at ventricular depolarization's end. The QRS complex should measure ≤ 0.11 second (Fig. 6).

Heart rate can be determined by one of several methods. The first, counting the number of complexes in a 6-second strip and multiplying by 10, serves as an estimate of the

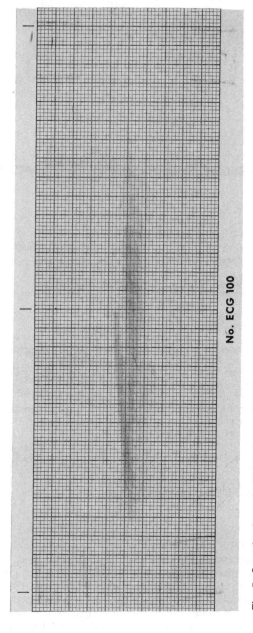

No. ECG 100

Fig. 5. Sample electrocardiographic paper with grids.

8

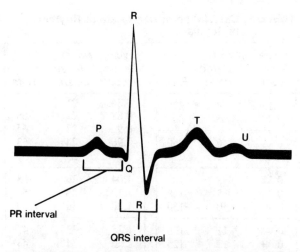

Fig. 6. Measurement of PR and QRS intervals. PR interval = number of small squares from first deflection of atrial depolarization to first deflection of QRS complex × 0.04. QRS interval = number of small squares from first deflection from baseline caused by ventricular depolarization to return to baseline at ventricular depolarization's end × 0.04.

number of beats per minute and may be used with both regular and irregular rhythms.

Each small square is equal to 0.04 second. Fifteen hundred small squares are equal to 1 minute (0.04 × 1500 = 60 seconds = 1 minute). A second method of measuring heart rate is to divide 1500 by the number of small squares between each complex (P waves if measuring atrial rate, R waves if measuring ventricular rate). Third, each large square equals 0.20 second. Three hundred large squares equal 1 minute (0.20 × 300 = 60 second = 1 minute). Therefore, divide 300 by the number of large squares between complexes to obtain heart rate.

Note: If rhythm is irregular, counting the number of squares in a single R-R interval will provide an *approximate* rate rather than the precise rate that would be obtained with a regular rhythm. For rhythms that are irregular, a range may be obtained by measuring the shortest interval between two complexes and the longest interval. You may wish to indicate average rate as well.

TABLE 1. Calculation of Heart Rate (If Rhythm Is Regular)

Cycle length (sec)	No. of 0.04-sec squares	Rate	Cycle length (sec)	No. of 0.04-sec squares	Rate
0.16	4	375	0.84	21	72
0.20	5	300	0.88	22	68
			0.92	23	65
0.24	6	250	0.96	24	63
0.28	7	214	1.00	25	60
0.32	8	188	1.04	26	58
0.36	9	168	1.12	28	54
0.40	10	150	1.20	30	50
0.44	11	136	1.28	32	47
0.48	12	125	1.36	34	44
			1.44	36	42
0.52	13	115	1.52	38	40
0.56	14	107			
0.60	15	100	1.60	40	38
			1.68	42	36
0.64	16	94	1.76	44	35
0.68	17	88			
			1.92	48	31
0.72	18	83	2.00	50	30
0.76	19	79			
0.80	20	75			

If the rhythm is regular, you might wish to make your calibrations from Table 1.

Basic Monitoring Leads

Although cardiac monitoring is not the final word in ECG interpretation, it does play an important and valuable role. Cardiac patients cannot constantly be confined to their beds with a continuous electrocardiograph running. Monitors allow patients more mobility as well as provide an ongoing reading of their hearts' activity. While we cannot depend on watching monitors for evidence of ischemia, infarction, and so forth, we can monitor-watch for early detection of cardiac arrhythmias. But, remember, monitors do not replace the 12-lead ECG, they only supplement. Because of the scope of this book, however, emphasis is placed on cardiac monitoring.

Many coronary care units (CCUs) have bedside monitors to which the patient is hooked, which also transmit to monitors in the nursing station. These bedside monitors have the capability of monitoring any of the 12 ECG leads, and have 5 electrodes for placement: right arm (RA), right leg (RL), left arm (LA), left leg (LL) and chest (V). These leads also are color coded for easy recognition: RA = white, RL = green, LA = black, LL = red, and V = brown. An easy way to remember lead placement is: "White is right with Christmas trees on the bottom, red going closest to the heart" (Fig. 7).

Many CCUs prefer to use five electrodes and to monitor the precordial (chest) lead V_1 because it provides the most valuable information about arrhythmias. The electrode for V_1 is placed over the fourth intercostal space, right sternal border. Lead V_1 represents electrical activity of the right atrium and right ventricle. Monitoring systems using three electrodes (positive, negative and ground leads) employ batteries to transmit to a central bank of monitors. Two basic hookups are used with these: lead II and a modified V_1 chest lead, or MCL_1 (modified chest lead). See Figures 8 and 9.

Through continuous surveillance, cardiac monitors and ECGs can provide invaluable information. They can help the coronary care nurse assess arrhythmias that require

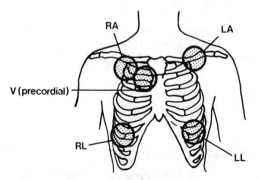

Fig. 7. Placement of five electrodes.

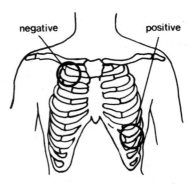

Fig. 8. Monitoring lead II. This is the hookup for a monitoring lead with an axis similar to that of lead II. In monitoring this lead, a sinus P wave is positive.

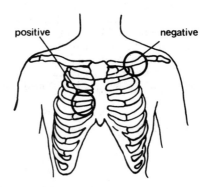

Fig. 9. Monitoring lead MCL₁. This is the hook-up for MCL₁. The negative electrode is at the left shoulder. The positive electrode is in the fourth interspace at the right sternal border. In MCL₁, a sinus P wave may be positive or negative.

therapy or even lifesaving measures. In addition, they can help one gauge effectiveness of therapy if one knows how to use them correctly.

Cardiac Arrhythmias

Cardiac arrhythmias generally are classified according to origin, mechanism, or both. By origin, we mean either supraventricular or ventricular. Supraventricular arrhythmias originate above the ventricle, in the S-A node, atrial myocardium, or A-V junctional area. Ventricular arrhythmias, as may be concluded by name, originate from the ventricles.

By mechanism, we mean the following:

Bradycardia: ventricular rate less than 60 per minute
Tachycardia: ventricular rate greater than 100 per minute
Block: improper or inhibited conduction

In analyzing each rhythm, the following steps should be used:

1. Determine ventricular rate
2. Measure width of QRS complex
3. Find P wave
4. Measure PR interval
5. Measure R-R interval
6. Look for beats that are different

Supraventricular

Arrhythmias

Sinoatrial Arrhythmias

Sinoatrial (S-A) arrhythmias generally are due to a predominance of the sympathetic or parasympathetic system over the S-A node. Included are sinus bradycardia, sinus tachycardia, sinus arrhythmia and sinus arrest (sinus pause).

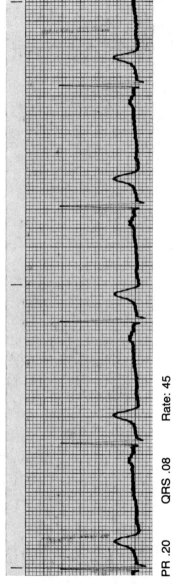

SINUS BRADYCARDIA

PR .20   QRS .08   Rate: 45

SINUS BRADYCARDIA

Mechanism:

Slowed rate of discharge of S-A node with normal conduction through A-V node and ventricles.

ECG Characteristics:

Rate: Less than 60
QRS: Normal
P wave: Precedes each QRS
PR interval: Normal
R-R interval: Regular

Causes:

Excess vagal stimulation
Sedatives; vagotonic drugs
Hypothyroidism
Myocardial infarction
Cardiac fibrosis

Significance:

Normal in healthy, athletic young persons. May lead to decreased cardiac output in patients with myocardial infarction. May permit escape of ectopic beats. Rarely causes syncope.

Treatment:

Generally none if rate is greater than 50 per minute or patient is asymptomatic.

Drug therapy if rate becomes critical, *i.e.,* if symptoms of inadequate cardiac output or ectopic beats occur.

- Atropine 0.5 to 1 mg IV push. May repeat every 5 minutes to 2 . Up to 5 to 10 mg may be used if necessary. (*Note:* doses less than 0.5 mg can cause more severe bradycardia.) Contraindicated with patients having wide or open angle glaucoma.
- Isuprel 1 mg/500 cc D5W IV infusion at rate of 1 to 5 μg/minute. Used when atropine is contraindicated. Relatively contraindicated in acute myocardial infarction.

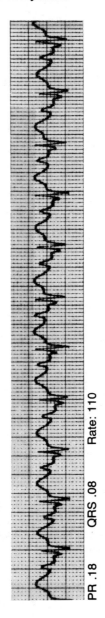

SINUS TACHYCARDIA

PR .18   QRS .08   Rate: 110

SINUS TACHYCARDIA

Mechanism:

Increased rate of discharge of S-A node, generally with normal conduction through A-V node and ventricles.

ECG Characteristics:

Rate: Greater than 100 (but usually not above 150)
QRS: Usually normal
P wave: Precedes each QRS complex
PR interval: Usually normal
R-R interval: Regular

Causes:

Excess sympathetic stimulation
Emotional reactions, *e.g.,* fear, anxiety, joy
Hypothension
Fever
Hypoxia
Hyperthyroidism
Drugs, *e.g.,* sympathomimetics, vagolytics

Significance:

Normal physiologic compensatory mechanism. Well tolerated by healthy persons. In patients with damaged hearts, may produce angina and inadequate cardiac output.

Treatment of Underlying Cause:

Inderal if condition is due to hyperthyroidism (Graves' disease); elevated heart rate is one of the signs patients with hyperthyroidism display. The dosage is as follows: Inderal 1 to 3 mg/50 cc D5W or NS infused slowly, not to exceed 1 mg/minute. After initial infusion, another dose may be given in 2 minutes. Subsequent doses are usually given no sooner than every 4 hours. Usual maintenance dosage is 10 to 80 mg. p.o.q. 6 to 8 hours. (*Note:* Severe bradycardia and/or heart block may occur with first dose. Preferably should be administered with physician monitoring.) *Nursing Action:* Check B.P. and apical pulse rate before giving Inderal. If extremes in pulse rate are detected, withhold drug and immediately notify physician. (See treatment for severe bradycardia if it develops.) Double-check dose and route. IV doses are much smaller than p.o. doses.

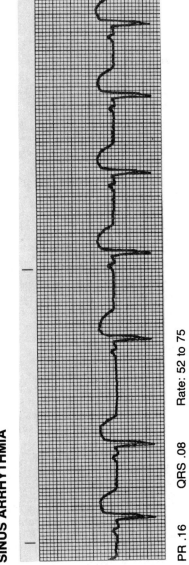

SINUS ARRHYTHMIA

PR .16   QRS .08   Rate: 52 to 75

SINUS ARRHYTHMIA

Mechanism:

Generally a reflex variation of vagal tone with respiration, *i.e.*, increases with inspiration and decreases with expiration, while conduction generally remains normal.

ECG Characteristics:

Rate: Generally 60 to 100
QRS: Usually normal
P wave: Present before each QRS
PR interval: Normal and regular
R-R interval: Irregular (phasic variation in cycle length of greater than 0.16 seconds)

Cause:

Varying vagal stimulation

Significance:

Normally found in healthy children and young adults. May be found frequently in healthy elderly adults. No problem arises unless rate becomes very slow.

Treatment:

Generally none.
Exercise or drugs may be used to increase heart rate and alleviate sinus arrhythmia.
If heart rate becomes too slow, treatment is same as in sinus bradycardia.

SINUS ARREST (SINUS PAUSE)

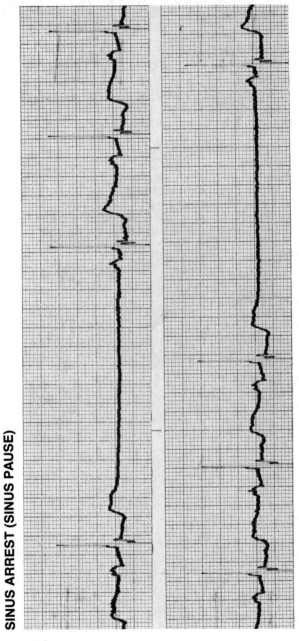

PR .28   QRS .08   Rate 54

Sinus bradycardia with first-degree A-V block. Two periods of sinus arrest, one lasting 3.16 seconds and one lasting

22

SINUS ARREST (SINUS PAUSE)

Mechanism:

S-A node fails to emit one or more impulses. Normal sinus rhythm usually is resumed after one or more beats have been missed. If S-A node fails for prolonged period, a junctional or ventricular pacemaker may take over. If this fails to occur, cardiac standstill ensues.

ECG Characteristics:

Rate: May occur at any rate
QRS: None seen during period of arrest
P wave: By definition, none seen during period of arrest
R-R interval: Irregular

Causes:

Rarely occurs in healthy individuals.
Increased vagal stimulation due to drugs, *etc.*
Digitalis toxicity
Degenerative forms of fibrosis
Inflammation of sinus node or sinus node artery
Myocardial infarction (usually inferior) involving sinus node or sinus node artery

Significance:

Periods of sinus arrest may be associated with "sick sinus" syndrome. In this disorder, periods of sinus arrest may alternate with periods of atrial tachycardia. This poses a problem, since drugs used to suppress arrhythmia may lead to sinus arrest, and drugs used to correct sinus arrest may precipitate tachycardia. Such patients are usually treated by a combination of drugs (to slow the ventricular rate during the supraventricular tachycardia) and permanent demand pacemaker implantation (in order to avoid the slow rate when the tachycardia terminates).

Treatment:

If digitalis toxicity is suspected, discontinue the drug.
Atropine 0.5 mg IV initially. May repeat every 5 minutes to a maximum of 2 mg. (Remember, doses less than 0.5 mg can cause more severe bradycardia. And, as you may recall, atropine is contraindicated with patients having wide or open angle glaucoma.)

In cases where atropine is contraindicated, Isuprel 1 mg/500cc D5W IV infusion at rate of 1 to 2 µg/minute may be tried as the first therapeutic approach.

A temporary pacemaker may be used if patient is symptomatic and underlying cause is known and can eventually be alleviated. A permanent pacemaker is indicated if patient is symptomatic and underlying cause cannot be removed.

Atrial Arrhythmias

In an atrial arrhythmia, an ectopic focus in the atrial myocardium reaches its threshold potential and depolarizes automatically before a stimulus arising from the S-A node has an opportunity to depolarize it. Since the heart follows its fastest pacemaker, such ectopic impulses generally depolarize the entire heart.

Ectopic atrial impulse formation may occur in very rapid sequence, up to 500 to 600 times/minute, and conduction of all impulses to the ventricles would have disastrous results. The A-V node assumes a protective role by transmitting only some of these impulses to the ventricles. Ventricular rates, under these circumstances, will depend on refractoriness of the A-V node. Normally, atrial rates of up to 170 to 200 are readily conducted to the ventricles. Higher rates are conducted with greater degrees of block.

PREMATURE ATRIAL CONTRACTION (PAC)

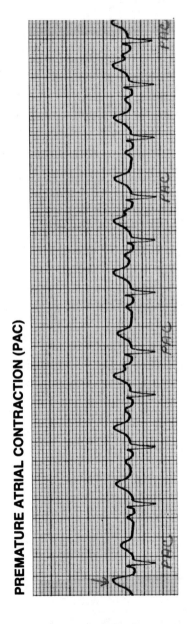

PR .16   QRS .06   Rate: 104

Sinus Tachycardia with PACs.

PREMATURE ATRIAL CONTRACTION (PAC)

Mechanism:

Ectopic focus discharges premature impulse which is conducted through the entire heart; conduction through the A-V node and ventricles is usually normal. PACs have a premature P wave with a contour similar, but not identical, to the sinus P wave and a PR interval greater than 0.12 second. If the A-V junction has sufficiently repolarized to conduct normally, and the ventricles have not completely repolarized, the supraventricular QRS may be aberrant in configuration.

A PAC may occur so soon following the previous beat that ventricular repolarization is not complete and the ventricles are refractory to depolarizing excitation. The premature atrial impulse then is dissipated within the conduction pathways and a ventricular complex does not follow. Such a nonconducted ectopic beat is called dropped or blocked. It is identified by the appearance of an early P wave of abnormal configuration without a subsequent QRS complex. When blocked PACs occur frequently, one has to take care not to confuse them with heart block because they can mimic this phenomenon.

ECG Characteristics:

Rate: Variable
QRS: Usually normal
P wave: Occurs prematurely, *i.e.,* interval between P waves is shorter than in normal cycle. Shape of premature P wave may differ from that of sinus P wave. P wave precedes each QRS (except with blocked PACs), but may be hidden in the T wave of preceding cycle.
PP interval: May be normal, shorter, or longer than in normal cycle.
R-R interval: Irregular

Causes:

May be seen in some individuals with normal hearts due to use of such stimulants as coffee, alcohol, tobacco, *etc.*
Mechanical irritation of atria due to atrial overload caused by heart failure or pulmonary embolism
Drug toxicity
Pericardial disease
Chronic obstructive pulmonary disease (COPD)

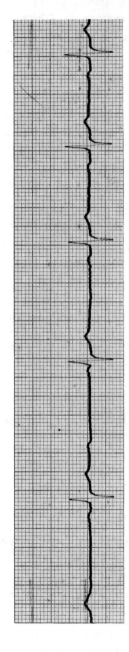

PR .22   QRS .10   Rate: 60
Normal sinus rhythm with 1° AVB and two dropped PACs.

Significance:

Usually benign in healthy individuals. May precede more serious arrhythmias in patients with heart disease.

Treatment:

If infrequent, no treatment is necessary.

If frequent, omission of irritants; sedation.

If drug toxicity is suspected, omit offending drug.

If frequent PACs occur with patients having heart disease, drug therapy is initiated:

- Digoxin: Loading dose 0.5 to 1 mg IV or p.o. in divided doses over 24-hour period. Maintenance dose: 0.125 to 0.5 mg IV or p.o. daily. (Average: 0.25 mg) *Nursing Action:* Check apical pulse before administering. Most physicians will note minimum rate for which digitalis is to be given; if not, hold the dose if apical pulse is under 60 per minute and notify the doctor. You may wish to request that he provide you with minimum pulse rate for the future.
- Quinidine sulfate or equivalent base: 200 to 300 mg p.o. every 2 to 3 hours for 5 to 8 doses with daily increases until normal sinus rhythm is restored or toxic effects develop. Maximum dose: 3 to 4 Gm/day. (*Note:* Quinidine should usually be administered after digitalization in order to avoid increasing A-V conduction.) *Nursing Action:* Monitor for signs of drug toxicity. Monitor quinidine levels.
- Procainamide HCl (Pronestyl, Procan, Procan SR, Pronestyl SR): used with atrial arrhythmias when unresponsive to quinidine. Dosage: 1 to 1.25 Gm p.o. If arrhythmias persist after 1 hour, give additional 750 mg. If there is no change, physician may order 500 mg every 2 hours until arrhythmias abate or side-effects appear. Maintenance dose: 500 mg to 1 Gm every 4 to 6 hours. *Nursing Action:* Monitor for signs of drug toxicity. Monitor drug levels.

PAROXYSMAL ATRIAL TACHYCARDIA (PAT)
(continuous strip)

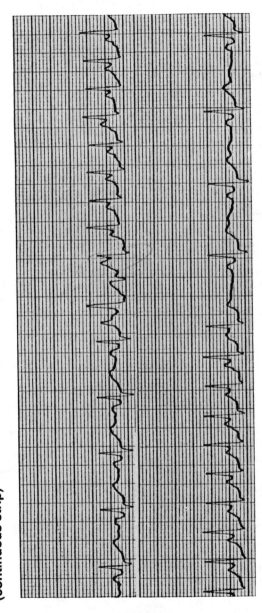

(1) Normal sinus rhythm: PR .14   QRS .08   ARVR 100→
(2) PACs→

(3) Paroxysmal atrial tachycardia with VR 188→   ARVR 79
(4) Normal sinus rhythm: PR .14   QRS .08

PAROXYSMAL ATRIAL TACHYCARDIA (PAT)

Mechanism:

Initiated by a typical PAC. Repetitive discharges from an excited region of the atrium result in a sustained ectopic rhythm. Beats of the tachycardia are precisely regular. Close to end of paroxysm, atrial beats become slightly irregular; then normal sinus rhythm resumes. There is some variation in the terminal portion of the QRS complex during the tachycardia; this is due to altered ventricular conduction caused by increased rate.

ECG Characteristics:

Rate: 140 to 220
QRS: Usually normal, but there may be some variation in terminal portion of QRS during tachycardia
P wave: Precedes QRS, but may not be identifiable
PR interval: May not be identifiable
R-R interval: Regular

Causes:

May occur in adults with normal hearts, especially in those under physical or emotional stress, or in those who use irritants such as coffee and smoking.
Thyrotoxicosis
May occur with heart disease, often coronary artery disease.
PAT with 2 : 1 A-V block is frequently seen with digitalis toxicity.

Significance:

May cause feelings ranging from palpitations, nervousness, and anxiety to dyspnea, angina, ischemic pain, and syncope. May lead to congestive heart failure (CHF) and/or hypotension in patients with heart disease.

Treatment:

May terminate spontaneously in normal healthy patients.
Vagal stimulation: Valsalva maneuver, carotid sinus massage, diving reflex, and gagging serve as the first line of therapy, either terminating PAT or leaving it unaffected (slight slowing may occur during vagal stimulation). Such

maneuvers should be tried by physician after each pharmacologic approach.

Oxygen if required for S.O.B.

Maintenance of an open vein, either by means of KVO-IV or heparin lock.

If digitalis toxicity is suspected, stop this medication and correct hypokalemia if present.

Verapamil 4 to 10 mg (0.075 to 0.15 mg/kg) IV push over 60 seconds with ECG and B.P. monitoring. Dose may be repeated in 30 minutes if there is no response. Bolus injection may be followed with maintenance infusion of 0.005 mg/kg/minute. Starting oral dose is 80 mg every 6 to 8 hours. Dosage may be increased by weekly intervals. Some patients may require up to 480 mg daily. Patients with severely compromised cardiac function or those who are receiving beta blockers should receive lower doses of verapamil. These patients should be monitored very closely. In older patients, IV doses should be administered over at least 3 minutes in order to minimize risk of adverse effects.

General Nursing Actions: Notify physician if signs of CHF occur, *e.g.,* swelling of hands and feet, shortness of breath, rales auscultated in lungs.

If the above approaches are unsuccessful, IV digitalis administration may be attempted next: digoxin 0.5 to 1 mg IV, followed by 0.25 mg every 2 to 4 hours, with the total dose being less than 1.5 mg within a 24-hour period. Oral digitalis administration to terminate an acute attack of PAT is generally not indicated. Vagal maneuvers previously ineffectual may terminate PAT following digitalis, and therefore should be repeated.

Inderal (propranolol) may be attempted if digitalis administration is unsuccessful. The usual dosage is 0.5 to 1 mg per minute IV for a total dose of 0.5 to 3 mg. (*Note:* Use cautiously in patients with heart failure or chronic lung disease because of the possibility of bronchospasm.)

Pressors, *e.g.,* tensilon or phenylephrine, may be used.

Electric cardioversion should be attempted, particularly if the patient shows signs or symptoms of cardiac decompensation. If digitalis or propranolol have been given, cardioversion is relatively contraindicated because of a likelihood of post-shock ventricular arrhythmias.

Pronestyl, quinidine, or Norpace may be required to terminate PAT in some patients; however, these drugs are more often given to prevent recurrences.

ATRIAL TACHYCARDIA WITH BLOCK

Mechanism:

Probably circus rhythm. A-V node transmits every second, third, fourth, or variable impulse, producing atrial tachycardia with 2:1, 3:1, 4:1, or variable conduction ratio or A-V block.

ECG Characteristics:

Rate: Atrial—200 to 250 per minute, but can be slower
      Ventricular—variable
QRS: Usually normal
P wave: Normal-looking P waves with characteristic iso-electric intervals between them are usually present in all leads
PR interval: Not seen
R-R interval: Usually regular, but atrial tachycardia with block may have an irregular ventricular response

Causes:

Digitalis toxicity
Significant organic heart disease such as coronary artery disease or cor pulmonale

Significance:

May lead to heart failure if ventricular response is rapid. May be a sign of left ventricular failure.

Treatment:

If ventricular rate is in normal range and patient is asymptomatic, no therapy may be necessary.

In patient not taking digitalis, atrial tachycardia with block may be treated with digitalis to slow the ventricular response. Loading dose: 0.5 to 1 mg IV or p.o. in divided doses over 24-hour period. Maintenance dose: 0.125 to 0.5 mg IV or p.o. daily. (Average dose: 0.25 mg)

Verapamil, because of its beta-blocking effect, may be used to slow ventricular rate. Dosage 5 to 10 mg IV push over 60 seconds with ECG and B.P. monitoring. Dose may be repeated in 30 minutes if there is no response. Bolus injection may be followed with maintenance infusion of 0.005 mg/kg/minute. Starting oral dose is 80 mg every 6 to 8 hours. Dosage may be increased by weekly intervals.

ATRIAL TACHYCARDIA WITH 2:1 A-V BLOCK

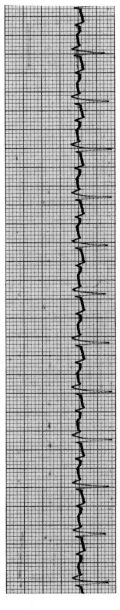

QRS .08   Atrial rate: 230   Ventricular rate: 115

Nursing Actions: With older patients, IV doses should be administered over at least 3 minutes in order to minimize risk of adverse effects.

Inderal may also be used for its beta-blocking effect.

If atrial tachycardia with A-V block persists after digitalization, oral quinidine, Norpace, or procainamide may be added.

Quinidine sulfate or equivalent base: 200 mg p.o. every 2 to 3 hours for 5 to 8 doses, with daily increases until normal sinus rhythm or toxic effects develop. (*Note:* Quinidine should only be administered after digitalization in order to avoid increasing A-V conduction.) Maximum dose: 3 to 4 Gm/day.)

Procainamide HCl (Pronestyl, Procan, Procan SR, Pronestyl SR): used with atrial arrhythmias when unresponsive to quinidine. Dosage: 1 to 1.25 Gm p.o. If arrhythmias persist after 1 hour, give additional 750 mg. If there is no change, physician may order 500 mg every 2 hours until arrhythmias abate or side-effects appear. Maintenance dose is 500 mg to 1 Gm every 4 to 6 hours. *Nursing Actions:* Monitor for signs and symptoms of toxicity. Monitor drug levels.

In some patients, this rhythm may resist termination by pharmacologic means. If digitalis excess is not the cause, cardioversion may be attempted.

Very slow ventricular rates might respond to atropine, 0.5 mg increments IV. (*Note:* Doses less than 0.5 mg can cause more severe slow ventricular rates. This drug is contraindicated with patients having wide or open angle glaucoma.

May require temporary pacemaker until underlying cause can be removed.

If atrial tachycardia with block occurs in a patient receiving digitalis, it initially must be assumed that digitalis toxicity exists, particularly in a patient who has recently received diuretics, who has a low serum potassium level, in whom digitalis dosage has been increased, or who has multiple premature ventricular contractions. In such cases, corrective measures include omission of digitalis and potassium-depleting diuretics and the administration of potassium chloride orally (30 to 45 mEq initially, repeated in 1 hour if necessary).

ATRIAL FLUTTER WITH 2:1, 3:1, 4:1 A-V BLOCK

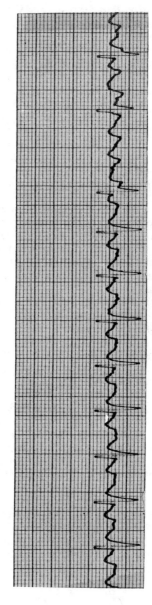

QRS .10   Atrial rate: 250   Ventricular rate: 70–150

ATRIAL FLUTTER

Mechanism:

Atrial repolarization is altered, changing shape of atrial wave itself. The wave tends to become bidirectional, and, at very rapid rates, atrial complexes take on a characteristic sawtoothed form, called F or flutter waves. Variable A-V conduction occurs when incomplete recovery and variation in transmission occur in the A-V node because of extremely rapid atrial firing rate. This results in changes in F-R intervals and contours. The A-V node transmits every second, third, or fourth impulse, producing flutter with 2:1, 3:1, 4:1 block.

ECG Characteristics:

Rate: Atrial—260 to 360 (usually about 300) per minute
       Ventricular—multiple of atrial rate

QRS: Normal

P wave: Normal P waves are not seen; instead, there are F waves that recur at a rate of about 300, producing characteristic sawtooth pattern.

PR interval: Not seen; instead F-R interval may be constant or varying

R-R interval: Usually regular, but atrial flutter with an irregular ventricular response may be seen; is referred to as "impure" atrial flutter. *Note:* When ventricular response is very rapid, it may be difficult to differentiate atrial flutter from PAT. Brief carotid sinus pressure will usually produce slowing of ventricular response so that flutter waves readily can be seen (done by physician).

Causes:

Arteriosclerotic or rheumatic heart disease
Myocardial infarction
Hyperthyroidism
Pulmonary embolism
Chronic obstructive pulmonary disease (COPD)
Congestive heart failure (CHF)

Significance:

May lead to failure if ventricular response is rapid. May be a sign of left ventricular failure. Usually responds to carotid massage with a decrease in ventricular rate in step-wise multiples and returns in reverse fashion to former ventricular rate at termination; rarely restores to sinus rhythm.

Treatment:

Verapamil (Isoptin) 5 mg slow IV push to slow ventricular response.

Digitalis to slow ventricular response (maintain resting apical pulse of 60 to 80 beats/minute, not to exceed 100/minute after slight exercise). Loading dose: 0.5 to 1 mg IV or p.o. in divided doses over 24-hour period. Maintenance dose: 0.125 to 0.5 mg IV or p.o. daily. (Average dose: 0.25 mg daily)

Propranolol (Inderal) may be used in combination with digitalis to slow ventricular rate when digitalis alone fails. Dosage: 10 to 80 mg p.o. t.i.d. or q.i.d. *Nursing Action:* Monitor blood pressure, ECG, heart rate, and rhythm frequently.

If atrial flutter persists following digitalization, quinidine 200 to 400 mg p.o. every 6 hours is used most often to restore a sinus rhythm. Maintenance doses are usually continued after reversion.

If A-flutter persists after digitalization and quinidine administration, termination may be tried with cardioversion and patient placed on maintenance doses of digitalis and quinidine after reversion to sinus rhythm. The usual initial energy level used is 50 watt-seconds. If shock results in atrial fibrillation, a second shock of a higher energy level may be used to restore normal sinus rhythm.

Sometimes synchronous cardioversion is initial treatment of choice for A-flutter. It promptly restores sinus rhythm with energy levels of less than 50 watt-seconds.

ATRIAL FIBRILLATION (A-fib)

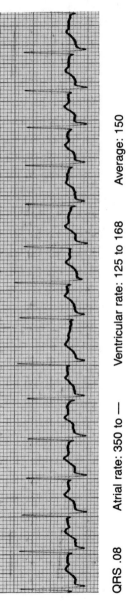

QRS .08 Atrial rate: 350 to — Ventricular rate: 125 to 168 Average: 150

ATRIAL FIBRILLATION (A-fib)

Mechanism:

Extremely rapid discharge of ectopic atrial focus. A-V node transmits impulses at irregular intervals. In untreated patients, ventricular rate is usually very rapid; it may drop as low as 50/minute in patients being treated with digitalis and those suffering from A-V node disease.

ECG Characteristics:

Rate: Atrial—350 to infinity
          Ventricular—variable
QRS: Usually normal
P wave: Not seen; usually irregular baseline is only evidence of atrial activity; tiny "f" waves can be seen at times, especially in lead V_1
PR interval: Not seen
R-R interval: extremely irregular ("irregularly irregular")

Causes:

Unlike A-flutter, may occur in absence of underlying heart disease.
Arteriosclerotic or rheumatic heart disease
Myocardial infarction
Hyperthyroidism
Pulmonary embolism
Chronic obstructive pulmonary disease (COPD)
Congestive heart disease (CHF)

Significance:

May lead to CHF. May lead to formation of mural thrombi. Cardiac output is reduced through loss of atrial contribution.

Treatment:

In absence of acute cardiovascular decompensation, digitalis is used to slow ventricular response (maintain resting apical pulse of 60 to 80 beats/minute, not to exceed 100 beats/minute after slight exercise). Loading dose: 0.5 to 1 mg IV or p.o. in divided doses over 24-hour period. Maintenance dose: 0.125 to 0.5 mg IV or p.o. daily. (Average: 0.25 mg daily) *Nursing Action:* Check *apical* pulse before

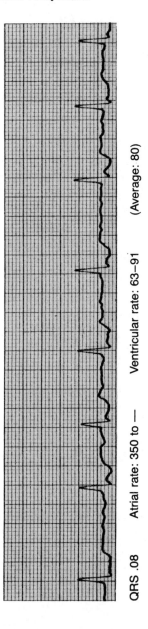

CONTROLLED ATRIAL FIBRILLATION

QRS .08   Atrial rate: 350 to —   Ventricular rate: 63–91   (Average: 80)

administration. If rate should go below 60 beats/minute, hold dose and notify physician.

Inderal (propranolol) may be used in combination with digitalis to slow ventricular rate when digitalis alone fails. Dosage: 10 to 80 mg p.o. t.i.d. or q.i.d. *Nursing Action:* Monitor blood pressure, ECG, heart rate and rhythm frequently. (*Note:* After long-standing A-fib, restoration of sinus rhythm may result in thromboembolism due to dislodgment of thrombi from atrial wall. Anticoagulation often is advised prior to restoration of sinus rhythm.)

Verapamil also may be used to slow ventricular rate. Dosage is 5 to 10 mg IV push over 60 seconds with ECG and B.P. monitoring. Dose may be repeated in 30 minutes if there is no response. Starting oral dose is 80 mg every 6 to 8 hours. Dosage may be increased by weekly intervals. (*Note:* With older patients, IV doses should be administered over at least 3 minutes in order to minimize risk of adverse effects.)

Quinidine together with digitalis administration is used most often to convert to a sinus mechanism. Maintenance doses of 1.2 to 2.4 Gm daily should be administered several days prior to planned cardioversion if the patient does not convert prior to then.

If sudden onset of atrial fibrillation with a rapid ventricular rate results in acute cardiovascular decompensation, cardioversion is the treatment of choice; begin with 100 watt-seconds, but usually higher energy is required.

WANDERING ATRIAL PACEMAKER (WAP)

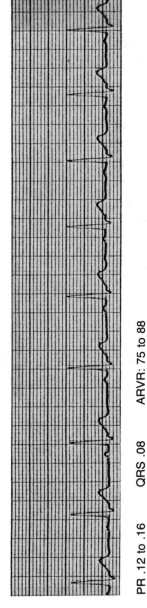

PR .12 to .16   QRS .08   ARVR: 75 to 88

WANDERING ATRIAL PACEMAKER (WAP)

Mechanism:

Pacemaker shifts from S-A node to various sites in atrial and/or junctional (nodal) tissue. Conduction through ventricles occurs in usual fashion.

ECG Characteristics:

Rate: Variable; usually slow
QRS: Usually normal
P wave: Changing configuration of P wave
PR interval: Irregular
R-R interval: May change slightly

Causes:

Excessive vagal stimulation
Sedatives; vagotonic drugs
Pulmonary disease

Significance:

Normally found in healthy young people. May be found frequently in healthy elderly adults. No problem arises unless rate becomes very slow.

Treatment:

Generally none is needed.

Atropine 0.5 to 1 mg IV push if rate becomes too slow. May be repeated every 5 minutes to a maximum of 2 mg. Up to 5 to 10 mg may be used if necessary. (Remember, doses less than 0.5 mg may precipitate rate slowing more severely). Contraindicated with patients having wide (or open-angle) glaucoma.

Isuprel 0.02 to 0.06 mg IV initially. Subsequent doses 0.01 to 0.2 mg IV; or 0.2 mg I.M. initially, then 0.02 to 1 mg p.r.n.

HIGH JUNCTIONAL BEATS

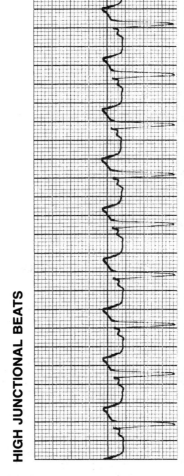

(Kelly SJ: ECG Interpretation: Identifying Arrhythmias: Review and Self-Study Guide, p 53. Philadelphia, JB Lippincott, 1984)

Atrioventricular (A-V) Junctional (Nodal) Arrhythmias

Atrioventricular (A-V) junctional (nodal) arrhythmias arise when the ectopic focus in the area of the A-V node depolarizes automatically. This may occur if impulses coming from the S-A node are unduly delayed or inhibited, causing junctional tissues to take over pacemaker activity for the heart. In this case, the junctional pacemaker will usually discharge at an intrinsic rate of 40 to 60 times per minute.

Irritation of the junctional tissues by hypoxia, myocardial infarction, or drugs such as digitalis may cause the pacemaker to discharge prematurely, *i.e.,* before a stimulus arising from the S-A node has had an opportunity to depolarize the junctional tissue.

Stimuli arising from the junctional area are usually classified as high, mid, or low junctional beats.

Mechanism of High Junctional Beats

Stimulus arising from junctional area is propagated in a retrograde fashion through atria, producing a negative P wave immediately preceding QRS complex. PR interval is short since some of normal delaying action of A-V node is avoided. Conduction through ventricles usually is normal.

Mechanism of Mid Junctional Beats

Stimulus arises from junctional area and is transmitted to atria and ventricles simultaneously. No P wave is seen, since QRS complex produces main vector of depolarization. Conduction through ventricles usually is normal.

Mechanism of Low Junctional Beats

Stimulus arising in low junctional area is transmitted to ventricles first, usually in a normal fashion, producing a normal QRS complex. This is followed by retrograde transmission of impulse to atria, creating a negative P wave.

MID JUNCTIONAL BEATS

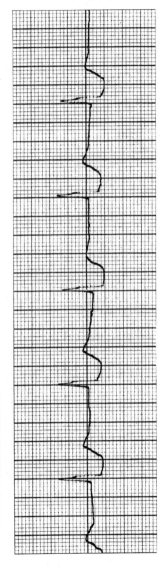

(Kelly SJ: ECG Interpretation: Identifying Arrhythmias: Review and Self-Study Guide, p 53. Philadelphia, JB Lippincott, 1984)

LOW JUNCTIONAL BEATS

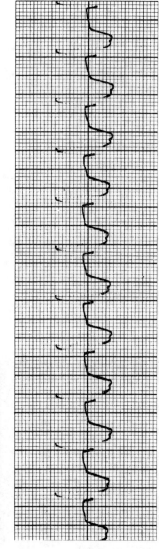

(Kelly SJ: ECG Interpretation: Identifying Arrhythmias: Review and Self-Study Guide, p 53. Philadelphia, JB Lippincott, 1984)

PREMATURE JUNCTIONAL (NODAL) CONTRACTION (PNC or PJC)

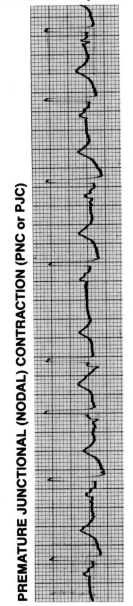

PR .16   QRS .08   Rate: 70

Normal sinus rhythm with three PNCs (PRs ranging from .06 to .11).

PREMATURE JUNCTIONAL (NODAL) CONTRACTION (PNC or PJC)

Mechanism:

Ectopic focus in junctional area discharges prematurely.

ECG Characteristics:

Rate: Variable
QRS: Usually normal
P wave: May be absent, may be upright and close to QRS complex, or may be inverted and occur before or after QRS
PR interval: Usually short (0.11 second or less) or may be absent or after QRS
R-P interval: Usually about 0.20 second
R-R interval: Irregular

Causes:

Disease or irritation of A-V junction
Depression of S-A node
Digitalis toxicity

Significance:

May precede junctional tachycardia.

Treatment:

Usually none. If drug toxicity is suspected, omit offending drug. If occurrences are frequent, treatment is similar to that for PAC.

Digoxin: loading dose of 0.5 to 1 mg IV or p.o. in divided doses over 24-hour period. Maintenance dose: 0.125 to 0.5 mg IV or p.o. daily. (Average dose: 0.25 mg.) *Nursing Action:* Check apical pulse before administering. Most physicians will note minimum rate for which digitalis is to be given; if not, hold the dose if apical pulse is under 60/minute and notify the physician. Request that he provide you with minimum pulse rate for the future.

Quinidine sulfate or equivalent base: 200 mg p.o. every 2 to 3 hours for 5 to 8 doses, with daily increases until normal sinus rhythm is restored or toxic effects develop. (*Note:* Quinidine should be administered only after digitalization in order to avoid increasing A-V conduction.) Maximum dose: 3 to 4 Gm/day. *Nursing Action:* Watch patient for signs and symptoms of drug toxicity. Monitor drug levels.

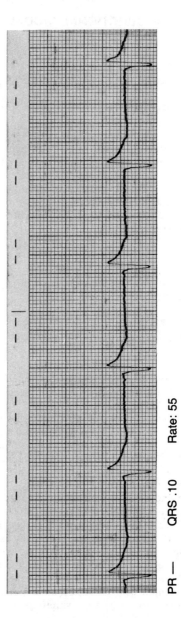

JUNCTIONAL (NODAL) RHYTHM

PR —   QRS .10   Rate: 55

JUNCTIONAL (NODAL) RHYTHM

Mechanism:

Slowing, blocking, or absence of impulses from S-A node allows a junctional pacemaker to depolarize heart.

ECG Characteristics:

Rate: 40 to 60/minute
QRS: Usually normal, but may be conducted with slight aberration
P wave: Upright and close to QRS; inverted before or after QRS, or absent
P-R interval: 0.11 second or less
R-P interval: 0.20 second
R-R interval: Regular

Causes:

May occur in normal individuals
May be due to organic heart disease, *e.g.,* rheumatic heart disease, myocarditis, or coronary artery disease
May be due to drugs such as digitalis or quinidine.

Significance:

In patients with heart disease, the slow rate may cause a drop in cardiac output. Slow rate may permit escape of impulses from a ventricular pacemaker.

Treatment:

Depends on clinical condition of patient; occasionally no treatment is required.

If due to digitalis toxicity, discontinue the drug. KCl administration may be required.

If due to slow sinus rate, atropine or Isuprel may be administered:

- Atropine 0.5 to 1.0 mg IV push. May repeat every 5 minutes to a maximum of 5 to 10 mg. (Remember: doses less than 0.5 mg can cause more severe bradycardia.) Contraindicated with patients having wide- (or open-) angle glaucoma.
- Isuprel 1 mg/500 cc D5W IV infusion at rate of 1 to 5 μg/minute (used when atropine is contraindicated). If slow rate sustains and patient is symptomatic, mechanical pacing may be necessary.

PAROXYSMAL JUNCTIONAL
TACHYCARDIA (PJT)

Mechanism:
Irritable ectopic focus in junctional area discharges more rapidly than S-A node, depolarizing entire heart.

ECG Characteristics:
Rate: 120 to 200
QRS: Usually normal
P wave: Inverted, before or after QRS, or absent
PR interval: Short or absent
R-R interval: Regular

Causes:
May occur in adults with normal hearts, especially those who are under physical or emotional stress, or who use irritants such as coffee and tobacco.
Is frequently seen with digitalis toxicity.
May occur with heart disease, often coronary artery disease.
Is a serious complication of myocardial infarction.

Significance:
May cause feelings ranging from palpitations, nervousness, and anxiety to dyspnea, angina, and syncope. May possibly lead to CHF and/or hypotension in patients with heart disease.

Treatment:
May terminate spontaneously in normal healthy patients.
Oxygen if required.
If digitalis toxicity is suspected, discontinue this medication and correct hypokalemia if present.
Verapamil 5 to 10 mg IV push over 60 seconds with ECG and B.P. monitoring. Dose may be repeated in 30 minutes if there is no response. Bolus injection may be followed with maintenance infusion of 0.005 mg/kg/minute. Starting oral dose is 80 mg every 6 to 8 hours. Dosage may be increased by weekly intervals. Some patients require up to 480 mg daily. *Nursing Actions:* Patients with severely compromised cardiac function or who are receiving beta block-

ers should receive lower doses of verapamil. These patients should be monitored very closely. With older patients, IV doses should be administered over at least 3 minutes in order to minimize risk of adverse effects.

ATRIOVENTRICULAR (A-V) DISSOCIATION WITH INTERFERENCE

Mechanism:

Ectopic focus in junctional area of ventricles discharges at rate faster than S-A node, depolarizing ventricles. Impulses are not carried retrograde to atria. S-A node fires at a slightly slower rate, depolarizing atria. An occasional sinus impulse may be conducted through A-V node and may "capture" ventricles; such beats may occur slightly prematurely, causing irregularity of ventricular rhythm.

ECG Characteristics:

Rate: Ventricular—variable
       Atrial—variable but slower than ventricular
QRS: Usually normal
P wave: Usually normal, occurring in regular rhythm, but may occasionally be buried in QRS or T wave.
PR interval: Irregular
R-R interval: Slightly irregular at times

Causes:

Digitalis toxicity
Organic heart disease

Significance:

Depends on rate; usually does not cause significant hemodynamic changes. May be forerunner of further arrhythmias.

Treatment:

If digitalis is implicated, drug should be discontinued, and administration of KCl may be required.

Ventricular
Arrhythmias

Ventricular arrhythmias are produced through automatic depolarization of an ectopic ventricular pacemaker. They may occur because of slowing or blocking of impulses arising higher in the conduction system. This type of impulse is called an escape. We are concerned primarily with ectopic impulses arriving prematurely, due to ventricular irritability, which may be caused by electrolyte imbalance, acid–base imbalance, hypoxia, drugs, or myocardial ischemia or infarction.

The output of the left ventricle supports circulation throughout the body. Ventricular arrhythmias may produce a very rapid decrease in cardiac output, and severe ventricular arrhythmias are immediately life-threatening.

PREMATURE VENTRICULAR CONTRACTION (PVC)

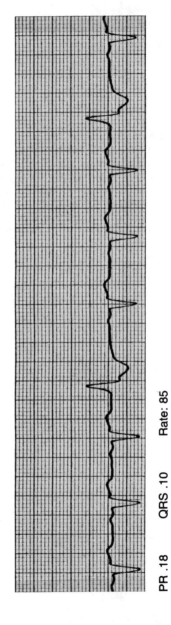

PR .18   QRS .10   Rate: 85

Normal sinus rhythm with PVCs in quadrigeminal pattern

PREMATURE VENTRICULAR CONTRACTION (PVC)

Mechanism:

The ventricular focus discharges spontaneously, depolarizing the ventricles. Since, in this instance, ventricular depolarization occurs through propagation of impulses from fiber to fiber, rather than through the conduction system, depolarization requires more time and produces a wide, bizzare QRS complex. The atria are not usually depolarized by this impulse, although retrograde conduction to the atria may occur.

The regular sinus impulse arriving at the A-V node is not transmitted to the ventricles, since they are now in a refractory state. However, the next sinus impulse is usually transmitted to the ventricles in the normal manner. This accounts for the "compensatory pause," so named because it results in no change in cadence of the previous rhythm.

A premature ventricular contraction (PVC) may occur without interfering with the normal cardiac cycle. This extra ventricular contraction is called an "interpolated PVC." Generally, it appears when the sinus rate is slow, and it allows the ventricles to recover from the "self-excited" beat in time to respond to the next sinus impulse. The PVC occurs between two conducted sinus beats. Because there is no retrograde conduction from the ventricles to the atria, sinus rhythm is not interrupted. After the PVC and the sinus beat that follows, major conduction pathways have recovered sufficiently to conduct sinus impulse to the ventricles.

ECG Characteristics:

Rate: May occur at any rate

QRS: Wide (0.12 second or greater); bizarre configuration totally different from normal complexes, but not necessarily oppositely deflected

T wave: In opposite direction from QRS

P wave: Not seen

PR interval: Not seen

R-R interval: Irregular; ectopic beat occurs early in the cycle and is usually followed by a compensatory pause (exception: interpolated PVCs)

PREMATURE VENTRICULAR CONTRACTION (PVC)

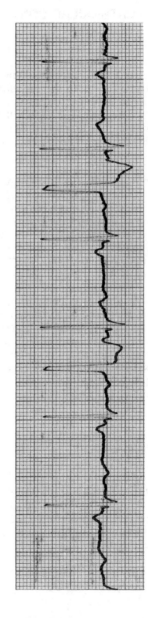

PR .17   QRS .08   Rate: 65

Normal sinus with interpolated PVCs (QRS .14)

Causes:

Ventricular irritability due to hypoxia, electrolyte imbalance, acid–base imbalance, myocardial injury, digitalis toxicity, or excess catecholamines.

Significance:

Occasional PVCs may occur in healthy individuals.

In patients with myocardial infarction, occasional PVCs may not be treated. Some physicians, however, may elect to treat the following patterns by administration of lidocaine or Pronestyl:

1. More than six PVCs per minute
2. Multiform (multifocal) PVC (usually more than five per minute)
3. PVCs falling on vulnerable part of preceding T wave (R-on-T phenomenon)
4. Ventricular bigeminy
5. More than three PVCs in a row (this is, by definition, ventricular tachycardia [V-tach])

It is wise to check your unit's policy and know what the physicians wish to have treated. Since this may differ from patient to patient, you may wish to have the physician specify his preference in the orders. If the patient has chronic PVCs, the physician may order "Treat V-tach only," or "Treat sustained V-tach only."

Treatment:

None in healthy individuals.

In acute cases, lidocaine is usually the drug of choice. Give 50 to 100 mg lidocaine bolus IV; may be repeated in 5 minutes if unsuccessful. Begin lidocaine drip at 2 mg/minute. Usual concentration: 2 Gm lidocaine in 500 cc D5W. Physician may order increase to 3 to 4 mg/minute p.r.n.

Pronestyl may be given instead of lidocaine. Usual concentration is same as for lidocaine: Pronestyl 2 Gm in 500 cc D5W and start at 2 mg/minute IV drip.

Dilantin may be used in treating digitalis-induced ventricular arrhythmias. Dosage: 250 mg IV over 5 minutes until arrhythmia subsides or 1 Gm has been administered. May be diluted in normal saline.

Hypoxia, hypokalemia and acid–base imbalance should be corrected.

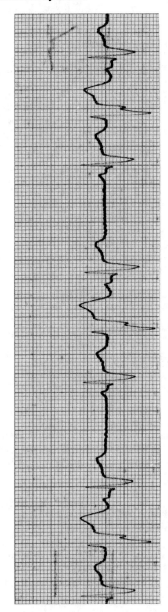

Ventricular trigeminy. (Note: PVCs are interpolated.)

In chronic cases, oral antiarrhythmic drugs may be used for prevention and control.

Procainamide HCl (Pronestyl, Procan) is used to eradicate PVCs. Loading dose: 500 mg to 1 Gm. Usual dose: 500 mg every 4 to 6 hours. *Nursing Action:* Blood levels should be noted at intervals if patient is on long-term therapy.

Dilantin may be used orally with a loading dose of 1 Gm during the first day, followed by 100 mg every 6 hours.

Norpace may be better tolerated by some patients than Pronestyl. Usual dosage: 100 to 150 mg p.o. every 6 hours.

Mexitil is presently an investigational drug with properties similar to lidocaine and is used when conventional oral antiarrhythmic agents are ineffective. Maintenance dose: 200 to 400 mg every 6 to 8 hours.

Tocainide is a major amine analog of lidocaine. Usual dosage: 400 to 800 mg every 8 hours p.o.

PVCs that are due to slow rate are eliminated by increasing rate with atropine or Isuprel, or by pacing.

Remember: Compensatory pause is one characteristic of a PVC. Although the compensatory pause can be useful in helping to distinguish PVCs from other arrhythmias, all PVCs do not have full compensatory pauses. When the PVC is sandwiched between two successive beats with no pause, you have an "interpolated PVC" (see pp. 00 and 00).

An Additional Note About PVCs:

In healthy persons without a history of ischemic heart disease, PVCs may be caused by anxiety, emotional stress, insomnia or insufficient sleep, nicotine, caffeine, and potassium-depleting diuretics. These PVCs are usually benign. Generally, they do not occur as frequently as in patients with ischemic heart disease; they are most often isolated; they usually are uniform (unifocal); and they rarely occur on the T wave of the preceding complex (R-on-T phenomenon).

ACCELERATED IDIOVENTRICULAR RHYTHM (AIR, "slow V-tach")

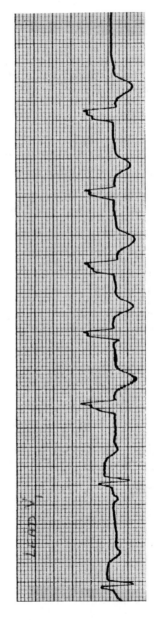

LEAD V₁

Sinus bradycardia with onset of five-beat run of AIR.

ACCELERATED IDIOVENTRICULAR RHYTHM (AIR, "slow V-tach")

Mechanism:

Ventricular ectopic focus emits impulses that depolarize the ventricles.

ECG Characteristics:

Rate: Below 100 per minute
QRS: Greater than 0.12 seconds; bizarre
P wave: Not usually seen
PR interval: Not identifiable
R-R interval: Regular

Causes:

Occasionally seen in patients with myocardial infarction.

Significance:

Does not usually have adverse hemodynamic effect.

Treatment:

Usually none is required.
(*Note:* deterioration of rhythm rarely seen; usually normal sinus rhythm is resumed spontaneously. *It is essential that ventricular response be counted so as not to mistake for V-tach.*)
Nursing Action: Elevate foot of bed so as to allow maximal cardiac circulation.

Life-Threatening Arrhythmias

VENTRICULAR TACHYCARDIA (V-tach)

Mechanism:

An irritable focus in a ventricle emits impulses at a very rapid rate, depolarizing the ventricles. This often is a re-entry rhythm.

The S-A node may continue to fire at its inherent rate, depolarizing the atria.

An occasional supraventricular impulse may arrive at the junctional area at a time when the ventricles have re-polarized after the preceding ventricular beat; in this case, the impulse arriving from atria may be conducted through the ventricles in the usual way, and a normal QRS will be seen; this is called "ventricular capture."

On occasion, an impulse of supraventricular origin may arrive at the Purkinje system simultaneously with an ec-topic impulse. The resultant depolarization of ventricles will proceed in part along normal pathways and in part through fiber-to-fiber spread; this results in a complex that looks partially normal and is called a "fusion beat." Occur-rence of a ventricular capture or fusion complex inter-spersed among a run of wide, rapidly occurring complexes is considered an important sign in identification of V-tach. At times, the rate of emission of ectopic impulses will become so rapid that no specific complexes are seen on the ECG. The needle records a fairly regular up-and-down swing called V-flutter, which is a close forerunner of ven-tricular fibrillation.

ECG Characteristics:

Rate: Greater than 100, usually 180 to 220 per minute

QRS: Wider than 0.12 seconds; bizarre (Ventricular complex in V-tach resembles configuration of PVCs patient had previously. Occasional complex may ap-pear completely or partially normal.)

P wave: Usually not seen; may be seen at much slower, independent rate, with no fixed relationship to QRS

PR interval: Not identifiable

R-R interval: Fairly regular

VENTRICULAR TACHYCARDIA

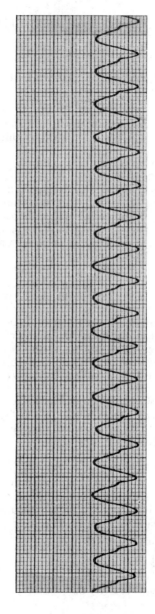

Rate: 168

Causes:

Most frequently seen in patients with myocardial infarction. May occur in patients with severe organic heart disease, Wolff-Parkinson-White (WPW) syndrome, digitalis toxicity, or severe electrolyte or acid–base imbalance.

Significance:

Rapid V-tach usually produces detrimental hemodynamic changes, due to inadequate filling and emptying of ventricles. May lead very rapidly to ventricular fibrillation and death.

Treatment:

Depends on patient's clinical condition.

If patient is unconscious and has no palpable pulse, initiate CPR and call a Code. Give 50 to 100 mg lidocaine bolus IV and begin lidocaine drip at 2 mg/minute (usual concentration: 2 Gm lidocaine in 500 cc D5W). Prepare for cardioversion.

If patient is found to be refractory to lidocaine, Pronestyl may be given in its stead. (Usual concentration: same as lidocaine—2 Gm Pronestyl in 500 cc D5W).

Inderal may also be used in cases of ventricular arrhythmia. 1 to 3 mg IV diluted in 50 cc D5W or normal saline solution infused slowly, not to exceed 1 mg/minute. After 3 mg have been infused, another dose may be given in 2 minutes. Subsequent doses may be given no sooner than every 4 hours. *Nursing Action:* Double-check dose, because IV doses are much smaller than p.o.

Dilantin may be used in treating ventricular tachycardia that is digitalis induced. Dosage: 250 mg IV over 5 minutes until arrhythmia subsides or 1 Gm has been administered. May be diluted in normal saline solution.

Bretylol is usually reserved for suppression of V-tach when conventional antiarrhythmic drugs such as lidocaine and Pronestyl are not effective. For IV drip, 500 mg in 500 cc D5W or normal saline infused at 1 to 2 mg/minute.

Remember: When patient is out of immediate danger, hypoxia, hypokalemia, and acid–base imbalance must be corrected.

VENTRICULAR FIBRILLATION (V-fib)

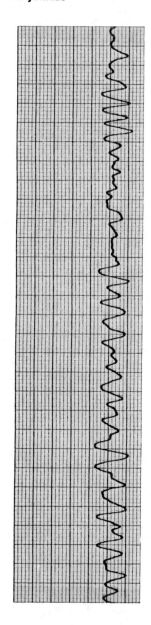

VENTRICULAR FIBRILLATION (V-fib)

Mechanism:
Rapid uncoordinated discharge of one or more ectopic foci.

ECG Characteristics:
Rate: Extremely rapid; irregular
QRS: No distinguishable complexes
P wave: None seen
PR interval: None seen
R-R interval: Not distinguishable

Causes:
Most frequently seen in patients with myocardial infarction. It usually occurs as a deterioration of ventricular tachycardia.

May also occur in patients with severe acid–base or electrolyte imbalance, as well as in patients with severe organic heart disease.

Significance
Immediately life-threatening. Patient appears clinically dead; biological death will ensue within approximately 3 minutes unless effective therapy is instituted.

Treatment:
Electric defibrillation starting with 200 watt-seconds; may have to increase to 300–400 watt-seconds.

Bretylol has immediate use in presence of ventricular fibrillation. For ease and speed of code team, it is generally diluted 500 mg in 500 cc D5W and rapidly infused as IV drip.

VENTRICULAR STANDSTILL (CARDIAC ARREST, ASYSTOLE)

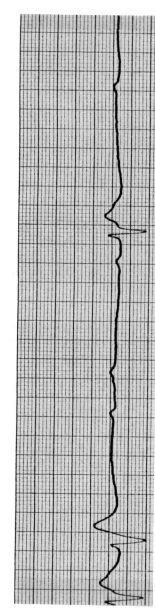

Some P waves are seen irregularly throughout as well as three "dying heart" complexes.

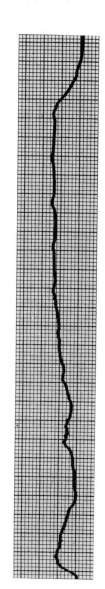

Another example of ventricular standstill or asystole.

VENTRICULAR STANDSTILL (CARDIAC ARREST, ASYSTOLE)

Mechanism:

No effective electrical activity is present in heart. Rarely, there may be atrial activity that is not propagated to ventricles.

ECG Characteristics:

Rate: Atrial—none or variable
      Ventricular—none
QRS: At times, complete standstill preceded by short, wide curves (referred to as "dying heart" complexes)
P waves: May be seen
PR interval: None
R-R interval: None

Causes:

Hypoxia from impaired respiratory function.

Respiratory impairment from anesthesia, anaphylactic reactions, hemorrhage, or drug overdosage.

In cardiac patients, it usually occurs at end stage of resuscitation or is preceded by marked, uncontrolled episodes of ventricular irritability.

Significance:

Immediately life-threatening. Patient appears clinically dead; biological death will ensue within 3 minutes unless effective resuscitation is initiated.

Treatment:

Immediate CPR
Electric defibrillation at 200 watt-seconds
Sodium bicarbonate ($NaHCO_3$) IV
Intracardiac epinephrine
Calcium gluconate IV
Vasopressors such as Aramine and Levophed
Transthoracic pacemaker

ABERRANCY

Normal sinus rhythm with aberrantly conducted nodal contractions.

ABERRANCY versus ECTOPY

Generally, aberrancy refers to those instances in which abnormal intraventricular conduction (bundle branch block) of a supraventricular impulse occurs temporarily. This isolated type of bundle branch block (BBB) occurs during rhythm that otherwise displays normal intraventricular conduction. According to Marriott, 80% of aberrancy takes on a right bundle branch block (RBBB) configuration.

Mechanism:

Aberrant ventricular conduction may appear in any supraventricular rhythm: sinus rhythm, nodal rhythm, paroxysmal atrial tachycardia (PAT), atrial fibrillation, atrial flutter, *etc*. Aberrancy depends on three factors: (1) unequal refractory periods of bundle branches, (2) critical premature impulse formation, and (3) length of the preceding R-R interval.

When unequal refractory periods of the bundle branches exist, an impulse initiated at a point of "critical prematurity" will encounter one bundle branch recovered while the other remains in refractory period. Thus, the impulse will be conducted down only one bundle branch, resulting in the bizarre QRS complex of BBB. Since the left bundle branch (LBB) is the shortest fascicle and normally recovers first, aberrant ventricular conduction usually assumes a RBBB configuration. If the impulse encounters both bundle branches in a refractory period, it will be blocked. An impulse occurring relatively late will find both bundle branches fully recovered and will be conducted in a normal fashion. Therefore, it is essential that unequal refractory periods exist for aberrancy to occur, and that such a phenomenon is favored by critically timed premature impulse formation (Fig. 10).

ECG Characteristics:

The most common form of aberrancy occurs when the cardiac cycle increases for one or more beats. Ventricular (QRS) complexes are normal until the heart reaches a "critical rate," at which time QRS complexes suddenly take on a wide, bizarre BBB configuration. As the rate decreases, the QRS complex generally returns to normal.

Critical rate varies among individuals. In patients with

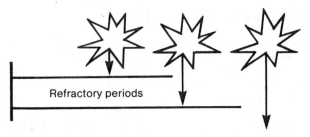

Fig. 10. Effect of unequal refractory periods on impulse formation. (1) Impulse encounters both bundle branches refractory; impulse is blocked. (2) One bundle branch is recovered while the other remains refractory; impulse is aberrantly conducted. (3) Impulse occurs relatively late and both bundle branches are fully recovered; impulse conducted in normal fashion.

badly damaged hearts, it may be comparatively slow. In other persons, a rate of 200 or more may be tolerated without aberrancy.

A well-known example of rate-related aberrancy is Ashman's phenomenon, in which a beat occurring shortly after a relatively long R-R interval is conducted in an abnormal or aberrant manner. The time required for repolarization is directly related to heart rate, *e.g.,* the longer the R-R interval, the longer the time needed for repolarization. When the rate is irregular and the impulse arrives relatively soon after a long R-R interval, portions of the bundle branch system have not completely repolarized; thus, the impulse is conducted aberrantly. This is the reason such phenomena occur so frequently in atrial fibrillation and atrial flutter (hence, Ashman's phenomenon).

With aberrancy of supraventricular impulses, we face a dilemma: Are the wide, bizarre complexes PVCs (and in need of treatment with lidocaine) or a premature, aberrantly conducted supraventricular beat?

We have already discussed the mechanism behind the phenomenon, following are a few measures that may assist you in correct interpretation:

1. *Check R-R interval.* It is never grossly irregular in ventricular tachycardia.
2. *Look for P waves.* Wide, premature beats immediately followed by P waves cannot be atrial in origin.

In general, when an independent atrial rhythm is evident in connection with a tachycardia having wide, bizarre complexes, the tachycardia is ventricular in origin. Remember, also look for hidden P waves.

3. *Check QRS configuration in monitoring lead MCl$_1$.*
   - RSR' pattern favors aberrancy. Remember, 80% of aberrancy has a RBBB configuration.
   - R waves taller than R' waves favor left ventricular ectopy.
   - LBBB pattern with wide initial R wave favors right ventricular ectopy.

4. *Analyze suspicious QRS position in cycle.* Tachycardia with wide, bizarre QRS that begins with a premature beat close to preceding normal beats' T wave usually are ventricular.

Treatment:

It is important to remember that it is infinitely more dangerous to fail to treat PVCs than it is to administer a lidocaine bolus to a patient having aberrantly conducted premature supraventricular beats. PVCs generally are the forerunner of immediately life-threatening arrhythmias and should be treated promptly. When in doubt, *TREAT.*

Heart Block

SINOATRIAL BLOCK

Mechanism:

Impulses are initiated by S-A node, but are not transmitted through atria because their spread is blocked by a "barrier" around S-A node.

If pause between conducted impulses becomes sufficiently prolonged, a nodal or ventricular pacemaker may depolarize spontaneously, producing a nodal or ventricular escape beat.

ECG Characteristics:

Rate: Slow or normal
QRS: Usually normal
P wave: Precedes each QRS complex, but one or more P waves fails to appear
PR interval: Usually normal
R-R interval: Irregular

Causes:

Familial or congenital (rare)
Infectious carditis after such diseases as diphtheria
Arteriosclerotic disease of S-A node, nodal artery, or right coronary artery
Degenerative disease of conduction system
Cardiomyopathies
Bursts of extreme vagal activity
Drugs, *e.g.,* digitalis, quinidine, Pronestyl
Scleroderma
May be associated with "sick sinus" syndrome

Significance:

Patient may be asymptomatic if it occurs only occasionally. When pauses are prolonged, syncope and Stokes-Adams attacks may occur. If no escape mechanism is produced, asystole will result. Escape mechanism may precipitate tachyarrhythmias.

Treatment:

If only occasional, none. If drugs are implicated, they should be discontinued. If there is excess vagal tone, vagolytics should be prescribed. If the condition persists and precipitates syncopal attacks, pacing is indicated.

ATRIOVENTRICULAR BLOCK

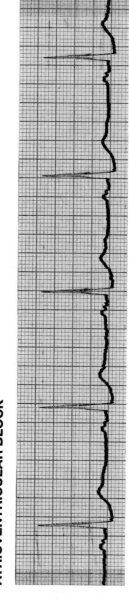

PR .24   QRS .10   Rate: 48

Sinus bradycardia with 1° A-V block.

ATRIOVENTRICULAR BLOCK

First-Degree A-V Block

Mechanism:

Impulse arriving from atria is delayed longer than normal in junctional area. Transmission through remainder of heart usually is normal.

ECG Characteristics:

Rate: Usually slow, but may be normal or rapid
QRS: Usually normal
P wave: Present before each QRS complex
PR interval: Greater than 0.20 second, but regular
R-R interval: Regular

Causes:

Rarely hereditary or congenital
Hypoxia of A-V node due to coronary insufficiency or
    myocardial infarction
Drugs, especially digitalis
Increased vagal tone
Myocarditis
May occur with premature atrial beats or atrial rates
    above 150 per minute

Significance:

If ventricular rate remains normal, patient may be asymptomatic. May serve as forewarning of higher-degree blocks.

Treatment:

If patient is asymptomatic, no treatment may be necessary.

If digitalis is implicated, discontinue the drug.

Ventricular escape beats occurring with slow rates normally disappear when rate is increased; they generally should not be treated with antiarrhythmics.

If a block occurs with rapid atrial rates, it represents a normal physiologic mechanism and does not require treatment.

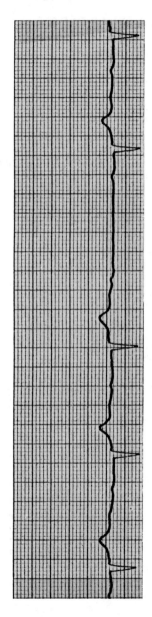

Second-degree A–V block: Mobitz I (Wenckebach)

Second-Degree A-V Block: Mobitz I (Wenckebach)

Mechanism:

Impulses arriving from atria are delayed for progressively longer periods of time until one impulse is not conducted to ventricles at all. This delaying and blocking action generally takes place in junctional area. Impulses that pass through this area generally are conducted in normal manner through His-Purkinje system.

ECG Characteristics:

Rate: Atrial—usually normal
　　　Ventricular—normal or slow, depending on number of nonconducted impulses
QRS: Usually normal
P wave: Precedes each QRS; occasional P wave not followed by a QRS complex.
PR interval: Becomes progressively longer until a nonconducted P wave occurs; then cycle is repeated. PR interval after nonconducted beat is the shortest.

Causes:

Rarely hereditary or congenital
Disease or impairment of A-V node due to myocardial infarction, hypoxia, *etc.*
Drugs such as quinidine, digitalis, Pronestyl
Hyperkalemia
Increased vagal tone
May occur with very fast supraventricular rhythms

Significance:

May be precursor of more advanced block. Slow rates may precipitate cardiac failure.

Treatment:

Unless ventricular rate becomes too slow, usually no treatment is required.

If necessary, atropine or Isuprel may be administered.
- Atropine: 0.5 to 1 mg IV push. May repeat every 5 minutes to a maximum of 2 mg. Sometimes up to 10 mg have been used. (Doses less than 0.5 mg can cause more severe bradycardia.) Contraindicated with patients having wide (or open) angle glaucoma.
- Isuprel: 1 mg/500 cc D5W IV infusion at rate of 5 μg/minute. (Used when atropine is contraindicated).
If drugs are implicated, discontinue.

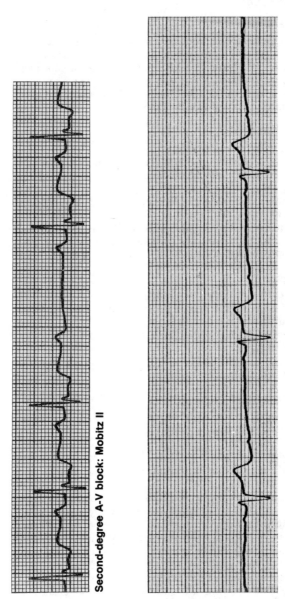

Second-degree A-V block: Mobitz II

Second-degree A-V block with 2:1 conduction ratio. *Note:* With 2:1 block every other impulse deriving from atria fails to be conducted to ventricles. At times, it is not possible to determine whether it is due to Mobitz I or Mobitz II block. Previous rhythm strips may provide the clue. Also note that one might conceivably confuse this strip with nonconducted PACs.

Second-Degree A-V Block: Mobitz II

Mechanism:

Impulses arriving from atria are conducted to ventricles usually with slight but constant delay until one impulse is not conducted to ventricles. Block may occur in A-V junctional area or, more frequently, in bundle branches.

When block occurs in bundle branches, impulses transmitted to ventricles usually are conducted by only one fascicle or branch. Totally blocked beats occur when this remaining bundle fails to conduct an impulse.

ECG Characteristics:

Rate: Normal or slow
QRS: Normal or wide
P wave: Precedes each QRS complex, but occasional P
    wave is not followed by a QRS complex
R-R interval: Irregular when impulses are not conducted.

Causes:

Rarely hereditary or congenital
Hypoxia or necrosis of parts of conduction system, due
    to myocardial infarction
Sclerosis of parts of conduction system
Drugs

Significance:

Mobitz Type II block is frequently the forerunner of a complete heart block.

Treatment:

If drugs are implicated, discontinue.
If patient has had recent myocardial infarction, transvenous pacing wire generally is inserted.

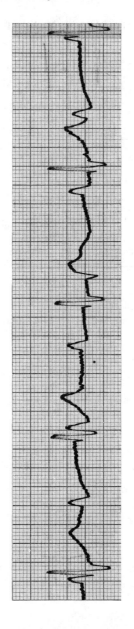

AR 72   VR 42

Complete heart block.

Third-Degree A-V Block: Complete Heart Block

Mechanism:

Impulses are emitted by S-A node and depolarize atria in normal manner, but none of these impulses is transmitted to ventricles because of block in A-V node, bundle of His, or bundle branches. Ventricular depolarization is initiated by spontaneous depolarization of an ectopic focus in junctional area or ventricles.

Note: There is no relationship between atrial and ventricular depolarization.

ECG Characteristics:

Rate: Atrial—60 to 100 per minute (usually)
Ventricular—30 to 40 per minute if ventricular pacemaker; 40 to 50 if junctional pacemaker

QRS: Normal with junctional pacemaker; wide with ventricular pacemaker

P wave: Normal P waves occur at regular intervals but bear no relationship to QRS complexes

PR interval: Completely irregular

R-R interval: Regular

Causes:

Rarely congenital

Ischemia or necrosis of A-V node or lower conduction system due to myocardial infarction

Sclerosis of conduction system

Drugs, especially digitalis

Severe hyperkalemia

Surgical heart block, *e.g.,* block that occurs following repair of ventricular septal defect.

Cardiomyopathies

Significance:

Cardiac output may decrease due to slow rate, causing heart failure, angina, syncope, hypotension, or Stokes-Adams attacks. Ventricular pacemaker site may become irritable and precipitate ventricular arrhythmias. Ventricular pacemaker may fail and lead to cardiac arrest.

Treatment:

If there is a stable nodal pacemaker, cardiac output is not seriously impaired, and condition is expected to be transitory, no treatment may be required. In most instances, however, the only satisfactory treatment is mechanical pacing.

In an emergency situation, Isuprel may be used until a temporary pacing wire can be inserted. Isuprel dosage: 1 mg/500 cc D5W IV infusion at rate of 5 μg/minute.

BUNDLE BRANCH BLOCK

Right Bundle Branch Block (RBBB)

Mechanism:

1. Septum is depolarized from left to right, as usual.
2. Left ventricle is depolarized, as usual.
3. Depolarization of right ventricle occurs late and slowly, since impulse must spread from left ventricle to right in a fiber-to-fiber fashion.

Anatomical Considerations:

The right bundle branch is the most vulnerable because

1. Being the longer, it requires a slightly longer period of time for complete repolarization.
2. Because it is long and thin, it is easily stretched by ventricular dilatation.
3. It has a single blood supply.
4. Its upper portion is near the intraventricular valves and may be affected by valvular disease.

ECG Characteristics:

Best diagnosed from precordial leads.

QRS: Wide; 0.12 seconds or greater

Tall, wide R' wave produced in right ventricular leads—aVr and V_1

Wide S wave produced in left ventricle leads—aV_1, V_4–V_6

In leads that produce R' waves, T waves are inverted

Causes:

May be congenital; on occasion, it is seen in otherwise normal hearts

Aberrancy

Ventricular hypertrophy

Acute dilatation of right ventricle, as seen in cor pulmonale or pulmonary embolism

Myocardial infarction

Lesions or surgery of tricuspid or, rarely, aortic valve

Degenerative disease causing sclerosis of one or more fascicles

Fibrosis of cardiac muscle, occurring most often near summit of intraventricular septum; may affect one or more fascicles of ventricular conduction system.

Significance:

RBBB per se has no effect upon cardiac output. It is only significant insofar as it aids in diagnosis of certain conditions.

Treatment:

If necessary, underlying condition is treated.

Left Bundle Branch Block (LBBB)

Mechanism:

May occur either with blockage of entire left bundle at its point of origin, or with blockage of both anterior and posterior left fascicles. In either case, ECG will present the same appearance.

1. Septal depolarization occurs from right to left.
2. Right ventricle is depolarized first.
3. Left ventricle is depolarized late and slowly through fiber-to-fiber spread of impulses from right ventricle.

ECG Characteristics:

LBBB is best diagnosed from precordial leads

QRS: Wide; 0.12 second or greater

　　　May be a small Q in V_1 and a small R in V_6, representing septal depolarization

　　　There is a deep, wide S in V_1 and a wide, usually notched R in V_6

　　　T wave in V_6 is inverted

Causes:

Almost any type of heart disease, including coronary artery disease, left ventricular hypertrophy, and congenital lesions involving septum.

Significance:

LBBB does not occur in normal hearts; its appearance is indicative of heart disease. LBBB per se does not cause reduction in cardiac output.

Treatment:

None for LBBB itself. Underlying condition may require therapy.

BLOCKS IN MYOCARDIAL INFARCTION

A-V blocks are relatively common in inferior wall (dia-phragmatic) myocardial infarctions. Why? The A-V nodal artery emerges from the posterior descending branch of the right coronary artery (90%) or left circumflex (10%). These blocks are generally transitory, being due to hypoxia of node rather than necrosis. Blocks are not nearly as common in anterior wall infarction, but if they do occur, they tend to be due to necrosis of the lower conduction system and thus are permanent.

Conduction disturbances increase the mortality rate in myocardial infarction. (Approximately 20% with inferior wall MIs and up to nearly 50% with anterior wall MIs).

Penetrating branches of the left anterior descending co-ronary artery provide the blood supply to the right bundle branch, anterior fascicle of the left bundle branch, and part of the posterior division of the left bundle branch. Obstruc-tion of this artery deprives a greater part of the lower conduction system of its blood supply, causing ischemia, necrosis, and loss of conduction.

Such blocks rapidly degenerate from first-degree A-V block to complete heart block (CHB) with serious hemo-dynamic consequences. In addition, myocardial irritability due to infarction often creates instability of the idio-ventricular pacemaker, and thus may lead to V-tach and V-fib.

Cardiac Pacing

Artificial cardiac pacemakers are electromechanical devices that deliver electrical impulses to the heart and stimulate muscular contraction. Originally, their only application was to keep the ventricles beating at a desired rate. Today, these devices have attained a high level of sophistication for their diagnostic and therapeutic uses.

Cardiac pacing is accomplished either by temporary transvenous pacing or permanent pacemaker implantation.

INDICATIONS

Temporary transvenous pacemakers are used both diagnostically and therapeutically. The major diagnostic uses for temporary pacing are to assess a patient's tolerance to stress created by rapid heart rates, and to examine signs of ischemia in patients with coronary artery disease by increasing heart rate by means of atrial pacing.

Therapeutic indications for temporary transvenous pacing include any transient and reversible situation, such as the following:

- Cardiac arrest
- Prior to insertion of permanent pacemakers or replacing pulse generators if the patient is symptomatic and emergency conditions exist
- To treat CHF in patients symptomatic to bradycardias and unresponsive to drug therapy
- Prophylactically in patients with asymptomatic complete heart block who are about to undergo general anesthesia for surgical procedures
- In the presence of bifascicular block with prolonged A-V conduction as a complication of acute anteroseptal wall MI
- To suppress ventricular ectopic arrhythmias related to slow heart rhythms and unresponsive to medical treatment

- As a precautionary measure following open-heart surgery
- For temporary symptomatic arrhythmias resulting from digitalis toxicity and hyperkalemia.

Permanent pacemaker implantations are done only for therapeutic reasons. Most commonly, permanent pacemaker insertion is necessitated by complete heart block associated with myocardial infarction. Even though the block may be transient, such patients, if not paced, may die suddenly within 6 to 12 months, presumably from a sudden recurrence of heart block.

Complete heart block creates symptoms caused by low cardiac output due to slow ventricular rate resulting in fatigue; congestive heart failure resulting in edema and dyspnea; and Stokes-Adams attacks (syncope), which are typified by sudden syncopal episodes resulting from a sudden arrhythmia such as ventricular fibrillation or ventricular standstill. Even asymptomatic patients should have permanent pacemaker implantation because these patients have a higher mortality rate without pacemakers.

Other reasons for permanent pacemakers include "sick sinus" syndrome (symptomatic sinus bradycardia); some forms of tachyarrhythmias such as paroxysmal atrial tachycardia (PAT) that cannot be controlled with drug therapy alone, and that have been demonstrated with temporary pacemakers in the laboratory to have been terminated by atrial or ventricular pacing to interrupt tachycardia; complete heart block due to fibrotic changes in conduction; and other symptomatic bradyarrhythmias including sinus exit block, periods of sinus arrest, carotid sinus syncope, and intermittent blocks.

ENERGY SOURCES

Lithium batteries are the most widely used energy source in cardiac pacemakers. Their expected longevity is 10 or more years.

Nuclear-powered pacemakers are rarely used because of governmental restrictions, prohibitive price, and the advanced age of most pacemaker recipients. The potential longevity of the plutonium source is 20 to 40 years.

No longer or rarely used are mercury–zinc batteries, rechargeable batteries, and biogalvanic batteries.

PROGRAMMABLE PACEMAKERS

Originally, pacemakers were set to deliver impulses at a specific, fixed rate and predetermined energy output. Once the unit has been implanted, no changes were possible. This is no longer true. A number of variables can be reprogrammed by noninvasive magnetic switches on current pacemakers.

- *Rate:* Pacemakers are generally set at a rate of 70 to 72 beats per minute for most patients. However, many pacemakers have a capability of adjusting the pulse-per-minute rate over a range of 25 to 125 pulse beats per minute. For example, a relatively slow rate of 50 to 60 beats per minute may be advisable for patients with coronary artery disease in order to reduce myocardial oxygen consumption.
- *Electrical Output:* Approximately 4 months following implantation of a pacing electrode, tissues around the electrode tip have normally stabilized. At this time, the pacemaker can be programmed to the smallest amount of voltage output that will still produce myocardial capture. By so doing, energy is conserved and longevity of the battery is increased. Along with reducing voltage output, *pulse width* is also reduced; minimum pulse width and voltage combined prolong the life of the battery. On the other hand, a pacemaker functioning well at the time of implantation may spontaneously fail to capture because of increased threshold caused by tissue changes around the electrode tip. In this case, the pacemaker's electrical output will be increased to resolve the problem.
- *Pacing Mode:* Some pacemakers can be reprogrammed from demand to fixed rate mode of pacing. With some of the more highly sophisticated pacemakers, both atrial and ventricular pacing and sensing modes can be reprogrammed.
- *Sensitivity:* Some pacemakers allow for sensitivity to be increased or decreased to meet patient's changing needs.

Other variables that can be reprogrammed include refractory period and A-V delay.

Reprogramming of the variables just described is done by use of magnetic units provided by the manufacturers.

The unit is placed on the skin directly over the implanted pacemaker. Activation of the programmer transmits the desired changes by means of a pulsating magnetic field to the pacer.

PACEMAKER MODES

The most important nursing responsibilities in relation to pacemaker patients are surveillance and evaluation of pacemaker function. In order to assess pacer function properly, one must first know what each unit is intended to do. There are numerous types of pulse generators available with a variety of pacing modalities, so many that it is impossible to describe each in detail. We will limit ourselves to general facts to assist in understanding pacemaker functions.

A number of demand modes have been developed since the first pacing units which pace either the atria or ventricles, or both chambers. Because of this, terminology has become complex, and one pacemaker might have several different names to describe it. Thus, in 1974 the Inter-Society Commission for Heart Disease suggested a three-letter code for identifying functional capabilities of pacemakers. In 1980, the code was revised by adding two more letters to describe programmability of pacemakers to control tachyarrhythmias. The three-letter code remains adequate for describing most pacemakers currently in use.

The first letter of the three-letter code indicates which chamber or chambers are paced; the second letter indicates which chamber or chambers are sensed. A = atria, V = ventricles, D = dual (or both chambers). The third letter describes the mode of reponse to sensed cardiac electrical potentials. T = triggered response, meaning the pacemaker will fire an impulse every time it senses cardiac electrical potential. I = inhibited response, meaning the pacemaker will *not* fire (*i.e.,* will reset itself) when it senses electrical potentials; it fires only in absence of cardiac activity. D = double, meaning both triggered and inhibited modes of response are in effect; the response is determined by the timing and sequence of electrical potential. O indicates that the pacemaker does not change its mode of function regardless of sensed electrical potential.

Artificial pacemakers essentially are of two types. The *demand (synchronous) pacemaker* delivers periodic electrical impulses at a given rate when the heart rate is slower than that set for the pacemaker. A special device shuts off impulses when the heart beats above that rate. The *fixed-rate (asynchronous) pacemaker* delivers constant electrical impulses at a preset rate regardless of the patient's heart rate.

Before one can properly assess pacing function of a pacemaker, it is necessary to know the purpose of a particular unit.

Asynchronous ventricular pacing (VOO) delivers a preset number of pulses per minute to the ventricles regardless of the heart's spontaneous electrical activity. It is rarely used; it exposes the patient to dangers of competition because most patients produce occasional intrinsic electrical actitivity.

Ventricular-triggered pacing (VVT) was the earliest used ventricular demand pacemaking. This type of pacemaker senses spontaneous ventricular activity and then fires. If no spontaneous ventricular beat occurs within a preset time period, called the escape interval, the pacemaker discharges at a regular rate corresponding to the escape interval. Although some of these units may still be in use, the ventricular-triggered pacemaker is rarely chosen today; its constant discharge of impulses hastens battery depletion, and all QRS complexes are distorted by this pacemaker's signal.

Ventricular-inhibited pacing (VVI) is most commonly used for temporary and permanent pacing. Spontaneous ventricular depolarization inhibits discharge of the pacemaker and resets the escape interval.

Atrioventricular sequential demand pacing is a dual-chamber pacing used with increasing frequency. It is used successfully in suppressing tachyarrhythmias with tachy-bradycardia syndrome, and with patients having a history of CHF who need "atrial kick" for improving cardiac output.

- *DVI mode:* Both chambers are paced sequentially. There is a programmed sensing and pacing interval of 0.16 to 0.20 second between atrial and ventricular pacing. Spontaneous ventricular depolarization which occurs within preset intervals senses and inhibits ventricular pacing. Spontaneous atrial depolarization is not sensed; the pacemaker continues to stimulate the atria at a fixed rate.

- *DDD mode:* Both chambers are sensed and paced. Pacing may be inhibited in either atrium or ventricle, or in both chambers. Most DDD models allow the patient a spontaneous rate from 50 to 130 beats per minute.
- *VDD mode:* Both chambers are sensed; only the ventricle is paced. Ventricular beats following closely after paced atrial beats are intrinsic and spontaneous. As the PR interval lengthens, a fusion between spontaneous and pacer-induced ventricular depolarization occurs. When PR becomes 0.20 seconds, the ventricular beat is paced. The ventricular portion of a pacemaker has a dual role: it is stimulated by atrial depolarization and inhibited by ventricular depolarization. Thus, PVCs would reset the escape interval.

To avoid errors that may lead to premature replacement of a normal pacemaker, certain rules should be followed to arrive a correct diagnosis:

1. Know the pacemaker's mode of function and anticipated signs of failure.
2. Inspect the long rhythm strip and select segments that have the most easily identifiable deflections.
3. Identify any unquestionable paced complex, idioventricular beats, and unequivocable P and T waves.
4. Use calipers to measure various paced intervals.

By means of these measures, it is possible to identify some of the unusual electrocardiographic phenomena seen only in paced patients.

ELECTROCARDIOGRAPHIC ABERRATIONS

Hysteresis: Following a spontaneous beat, some units may incorporate a slightly prolonged escape interval before returning to normal preset rate (Fig. 11). This normal phenomenon, called hysteresis, should not be mistaken for a broken wire or other false pacemaker inhibition.

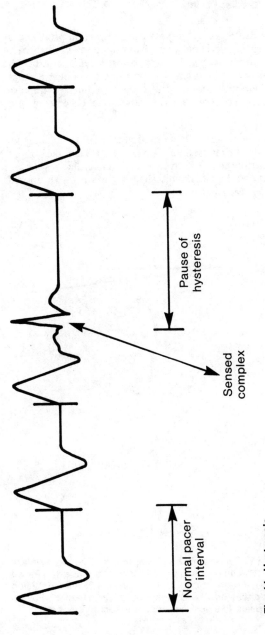

Fig. 11. Hysteresis.

Fusion Beat: A fusion beat is a contraction produced by merging depolarizing waves from impulses of both pacemaker and heart which begin almost simultaneously. The QRS is distorted, taking on a configuration bearing some resemblance to both intrinsic and pacemaker impulses (Fig. 12). Fusion beats occur with normal pacemaker function.

Pseudofusion Beat: In a pseudofusion beat, the pacer impulse is superimposed on the normal QRS complex, thereby distorting the QRS even though no cardiac response is elicited (see Fig. 12). This phenomenon is also seen with normal pacemaker function.

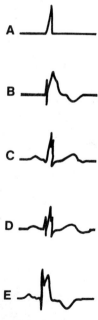

Fig. 12. (*A*) Pacer impulse alone; may not be seen unless pacemaker fails to sense or is in fixed rate mode. (*B*) Paced beat. (*C*) Spontaneous QRS complex. (*D*) Pseudofusion beat; spontaneous QRS complex is distorted. (*E*) Fusion beat; appears like neither paced nor spontaneous beat.

Tracking Pulse: A tracking pulse is a very narrow impulse of 0.15 seconds that is capable of producing a cardiac contraction. Several manufacturers produce pacemakers with this modification to permit easy identification of a sensed complex. This impulse will fall at the point in the QRS complex that is sensed. The only way this impulse can be identified with certainty is to know how the unit is designed to function and to observe that, despite the irregular spontaneous rhythm, the pacemaker impulse appears within each QRS complex.

False Sensing Failure: In false sensing failure, the sensing electrode detects the fastest-rising component of the intraventricular complex, which may occur later than the actual initial deflection, thereby giving the impression that the pulse generator has failed to sense the QRS complex. This phenomenon may be identified by noting that these complexes occur *only when the R-R interval is almost identical to the normal pacing rate.* Clearly premature spontaneous beats will not have a superimposed pacing impulse.

Many other phenomena may be seen with pacemakers. The more complex pacing units, such as the VAT and DVI, produce the more bizarre electrocardiographic aberrations.

PACEMAKER MALFUNCTION

Common causes of pacemaker malfunction include depletion of the battery, component failure, malposition of the electrode tip, and a fractured electrode.

Pulse Rate Drop

A drop in the pulse rate is often the first sign of pacemaker malfunction, particularly battery depletion. A rate drop that has a regular pulse is most likely caused by battery depletion. If the pulse is irregular, it is most likely caused by ectopic beats or by the patient's own rhythm competing with the pacemaker rhythm. Run a long rhythm strip when the pulse rate drop can be documented and notify the physician. The patient will need pulse generator replacement.

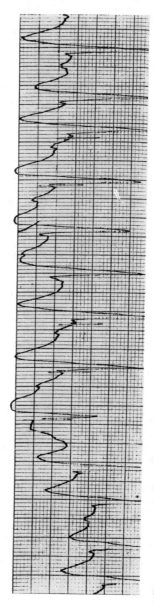

Runaway pacemaker firing at rate of 120

Runaway Pacemaker

Pacemaker impulses may occur more rapidly than the set rate, a phenomenon called runaway pacemaker. This is a most dangerous problem because accelerated firing can produce life-threatening ventricular tachycardia.

Causes:

Pulse generator malfunction.

ECG Characteristics:

Shows wide, bizarre QRS complexes, indicating ventricular tachycardia. Pacer spikes may or may not be present.

Signs:

Patient shows signs of insufficient cardiac output such as hypotension, increased heart rate, syncope, *etc.*

Nursing Actions:

Notify physician immediately

If indicated, call a Code and initiate CPR

Maintain constant surveillance of cardiac monitor and patient

Be prepared for immediate replacement of pulse generator or replacement of pacemaker

Failure to Sense

In failure to sense, pacing artifacts occur after spontaneous beats, within less than the preset escape interval.

Causes:

Malfunction of pulse generator

Lead displacement in myocardium

ECG Characteristics:

With malfunction of the pulse generator, pacer spikes are seen at inappropriate intervals. With lead displacement, no pacer spikes are seen even though the heartbeat is slower than the pacemaker's set rate.

Signs:

The patient usually shows no change in condition if the problem is due to pulse generator malfunction. The patient

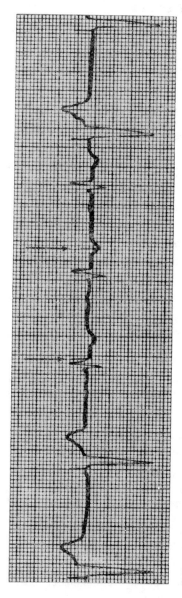

Failure to sense resulting in competition.

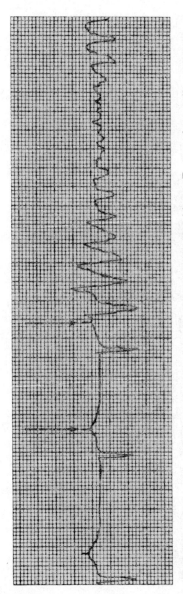

Another example of competition due to failure to sense: pacing stimulus hits on T wave of preceding natural beat, causing repetitive firing in the form of ventricular fibrillation.

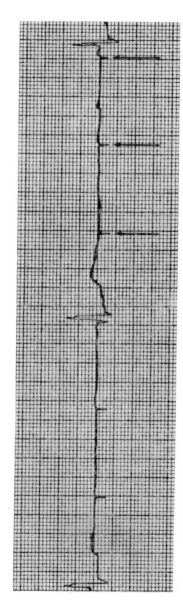

Loss of capture: small pacer spikes are seen but not followed by QRS complexes.

shows signs of his prepacemaker condition if the problem is due to lead displacement.

Significance:

Failure to sense exposes the patient to various arrhythmias. Competition may occur whereby the pacer fails to sense interpolated spontaneous beats, resulting in an increased ventricular rate, a potentially dangerous tachycardia. Ventricular tachycardia and fibrillation may result from a paced beat transposed on the vulnerable portion of the preceding T wave.

Nursing Actions:

Notify physician
Obtain 12-lead ECG
Maintain constant surveillance of patient and cardiac
   monitor
Be prepared to call a Code and initiate CPR
Be prepared to return patient to surgery

Loss of Capture

In loss of capture, pacing artifacts are seen but not always followed by ventricular depolarization.

Causes:

Weak impulse (low MA) from pulse generator
Lead displacement in myocardium
Electrode fracture
Dying heart

ECG Characteristics:

There are no pacer spikes, even though the heartbeat is lower than the pacemaker's preset rate. Smaller pacer spikes may be seen not followed by QRS complexes.

Signs:

Patient shows signs of prepacemaker condition.

Nursing Actions:

Notify physician immediately
Increase MA if due to weak impulse from pulse
   generator

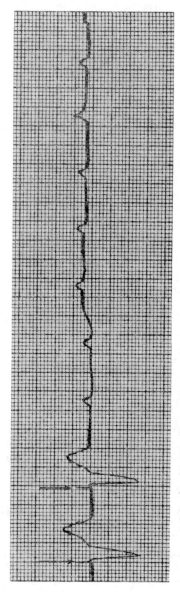

Failure to pace: only atrial activity from heart is noted.

Be prepared to call a Code and initiate CPR
Maintain constant surveillance of patient and cardiac
    monitor
Be prepared for pacemaker replacement

Failure to Pace

In failure to pace, no pacing artifact is seen even though the
patient's heart rate is below the preset pacer rate.

Causes:

Electrode fracture
Pacemaker failure

ECG Characteristics:

No pacer artifact is seen; prepacemaker heart rhythm is
seen.

Signs:

Patient shows signs of prepacemaker condition.

Nursing Actions:

Notify physician immediately
Be prepared to call a Code and initiate CPR
Maintain constant surveillance of patient and cardiac
    monitor

Other Malfunctions

A special problem with DDD pacemakers is that they can
mediate a pacemaker-induced tachycardia due to re-entry
impulse from ventricles to atria. When this is sustained,
serious tachyarrhythmias may result. Treatment includes
(1) turning off the power unit, (2) reprogramming the
pacemaker to another mode, and (3) administering
medications that suppress spontaneous cardiac activity.

Perforation of the ventricular wall by an electrode lead
also can cause pacemaker malfunction. In this situation,
the cardiac monitor shows no pacer spikes even though the
heart rate is slower than the pacemaker's preset rate. The
patient shows signs of his prepacemaker condition. The
patient may also have hiccoughs if the electrode is irritating
the diaphragm, or intercostal muscle contractions if the
electrode is touching them. A rare complication is cardiac

tamponade if the perforation does not seal itself. As with the previous pacemaker malfunctions, the following nursing actions should be taken: (1) notify the physician immediately, (2) maintain constant surveillance of the patient and the cardiac monitor, (3) call a Code and initiate CPR if necessary, and (4) be prepared to return the patient to surgery.

Defibrillation

Defibrillation is a lifesaving technique which involves application of electric shock to the heart in ventricular fibrillation. Ventricular fibrillation is due to uncoordinated discharge of impulses from multiple ventricular foci. This results in cessation of cardiac output. When sufficiently intense electric shock passes through the heart, all fibers are depolarized simultaneously and all intrinsic pacemaker activity is temporarily inhibited. Generally, the sinus node is the first pacemaker to recover, thereby enabling it to assume control.

If accomplished within a minute, defibrillation has a good chance of being successful. Since nurses generally are first to reach the patient's bedside, it is they who must assume responsibility for instituting defibrillation on their own initiative.

Technique of Emergency Defibrillation

1. As soon as ventricular fibrillation is noted on the cardiac monitor, take the defibrillator to the patient's bedside.
2. Confirm the diagnosis by checking the patient's carotid pulse; pulse will be absent. Usually, a glance at the patient is sufficient to determine if it is a false alarm.
3. Unless the defibrillator is battery operated, it must be plugged in and turned on in order to be operational.
4. Place electrode paste over the entire surface of the paddles, or place saline-soaked sponges in correct positions on the patient's chest. This is done in order avoid burns. Some manufacturers provide prejelled defibrillating pads.
5. Turn the intensity control to the desired watt-seconds level. For defibrillating an adult of average size and weight, 200 watt-seconds is recommended by the American Heart Association in order not to damage the heart.

6. Place the paddles on the patient so that current moving from one paddle to the other will pass through the heart. With anterior paddles, position one paddle near the right subclavian area and the other over the left precordium (Fig. 13). If a posterior paddle is used, place it under the left subscapular area, with the anterior paddle over the heart.
7. Firmly press the paddles flat against the skin.
8. Make sure no one, including yourself, is touching the patient or the bed. (Also, make certain the floor is dry under your feet.)
9. Trigger the current by pressing the discharge button(s).
10. Observe the shock's effect on the patient and on the ECG.
11. If necessary, reset the charge and defibrillate again. There is no limit to the number of times a patient may be given a defibrillating shock.

Remember, ventricular fibrillation causes clinical death and will result in biological death unless terminated promptly. Defibrillation is the most effective and success-

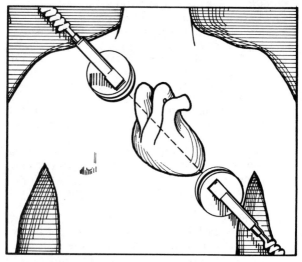

Fig. 13. Placement of anterior paddles.

ful means of correcting this lethal arrhythmia. All potential ill effects are immaterial in such a situation.

Defibrillation is also used to stimulate a heart in standstill. The electric shock may produce ventricular fibrillation, which then can be converted into an appropriate rhythm by a further shock. Although this procedure is not always successful, it is worth trying if other means fail.

Appendix I:
Antiarrhythmic
Drug Review

ADRENALIN, EPINEPHRINE

Mechanism:

Increases stroke volume and myocardial contractility.

Uses:

Direct stimulation of pacemaker cells during cardiac arrest. Elevates blood pressure when used in large doses.

Administration:

Given by way of intracardiac injection during cardiac arrest: 0.25 to 0.5 cc of 1 : 1000 solution. When given by IV infusion, dosage is titrated according to response: 1 to 8 μg/minute IV drip is usual.

Side-Effects:

Ventricular arrhythmias
Angina secondary to inability of damaged heart to meet increased oxygen requirement due to reduced coronary blood flow
Possible hypotension due to beta-adrenergic vasodilatation

Nursing Implications:

Monitor BP every 2 to 5 minutes until stable.
Monitor cardiac rhythm.
Watch for signs of overdose and discontinue immediately if any occur:

- Cold, diaphoretic skin
- Tachypnea
- Cyanotic nailbeds

ATROPINE (atropine sulfate)

Mechanism:

Blocks vagal stimulation to myocardium, increasing conduction velocity through A-V node.

Uses:

For treatment of symptomatic bradycardia and conduction defects of S-A and A-V nodes.

Administration:

0.5 to 1 mg IV push. Effect is immediate. (Doses of less than 0.5 mg can cause more severe bradycardia.) When given IM, effects are longer lasting, but less immediate than when given IV push; 2 mg IM is equivalent to 1 mg IV.

Side-Effects:

Dry mouth, pupil dilation, skin flushing
Inability to void in older patients, especially in men with prostatic enlargement
In presence of myocardial infarction, increased heart rate may cause PVCs or even ventricular tachycardia, though less likely a frequent occurrence

Nursing Implications:

Monitor cardiac rhythm and BP, and watch for PVCs.
Observe for complaints of urinary retention, bladder distention.
Maintain adequate hydration and oral hygiene.

BRETYLIUM TOSYLATE (Bretylol)

Mechanism:

Interferes with norepinephrine release at nerve endings. Inhibits uptake of catecholamines into nerve endings. Enhances myocardial contractility.

Raises electrical stimulation threshold for ventricular fibrillation. (Suppression of V-fib is rapid, usually within minutes of IV administration.)

Uses

Reserved for use in suppressing life-threatening arrhythmias when conventional antiarrhythmic drugs (lidocaine or Pronestyl) are ineffective.

Administration:

For immediate use in the presence of ventricular fibrillation, it can be administered *undiluted* at a dosage of 5 mg/kg by rapid IV bolus. If ventricular fibrillation persists, the dosage can be increased to 10 mg/kg and repeated at 15 to 30 minute intervals, not to exceed 30 mg/kg.

For IV drip, prepare Bretylol 500 mg in 500 D5W. Infuse at 1 to 2 mg/minutes. Usual IV bolus dose is 5 to 10 mg/kg given IV over 8 minutes or longer.

Side-Effects:

Hypotension preceded by hypertension (due to initial release of norepinephrine)

Transient occurrence of arrhythmias initially, especially in presence of digitalis toxicity

Nausea and vomiting

Adverse interaction with quinidine

Nursing Implications:

Keep patient supine until tolerance to hypotensive effect of Bretylol occurs. Tolerance develops unpredictably, but may be present after several days.

Expect vomiting after rapid IV administration of undiluted drug.

Monitor vital signs and cardiac rhythm.

CALCIUM (calcium chloride, calcium gluconate)

Mechanism:

Normal blood serum levels are necessary to maintain electrical stimulation threshold of ventricles for normal systole time and duration function.

Action:

Directly increases myocardial contractility strength

Is important to impulse formation of sinus and A-V nodes

Indirectly opposes action of potassium on myocardium

In elevated levels, contributes to digitalis toxicity effects (low levels do just the opposite)

Uses:

For cardiac arrest: 3 to 5 ml by intracardiac route of 10% calcium gluconate in solution enhances myocardial tone and adds strength to myocardial contraction.

After heart massage, with adequate ventilation: unsuccessful in improving heart tone, and ECG monitoring displays small amplitude fibrillating ventricular movements.

Administration:

IV injection of calcium chloride 5% to 10% concentration not exceeding 2 ml/minute. Calcium gluconate given in a 10% solution IV is less effective than calcium chloride.

Side-Effects:

Moderate hypotension by means of vasodilation.

Nursing Implications:

Continuous ECG monitoring is necessary during administration. Indications of hypercalcemia are seen as shortened ST segments, and Q-T intervals with bradycardia. Hypocalcemia expressions are prolonged ST segments and Q-T intervals, and shifting of T wave polarity, but duration of T wave remains unchanged.

Frequent monitoring is necessary for changes of normal serum calcium levels (8.5 to 10.5 mg/100 ml, or 4.5 to 5.8 mEq/liter).

ECG monitoring is necessary for changes in rate.

Caution should be taken with IV route to prevent infiltration, which produces sloughing of tissue.

Alert physician if patient is simultaneously receiving digitalis therapy.

DIGOXIN, DIGITALIS (Lanoxin)

Mechanism:

Increases ventricular contractility
Slows heart rate

Uses:

Effective in reducing heart's total oxygen demands; in heart failure, cardiac efficiency results from a reduction in heart's size.

To treat supraventricular arrhythmias, as in rapid uncontrolled atrial fibrillation.

Administration:

Parenteral digoxin, a popular digitalis derivative, is given in an initial dose of 0.5 to 1 mg, followed by doses of 0.25 mg every 2 to 4 hours until 1.5 mg has been given within 24 hours.

Another preparation of parenterally administered digitalis is lanatoside C (Cedilanid). It is fast-acting, but effects last only a short period. For maintenance therapy, oral route is common; dosage ranges from 0.125 to 0.375 mg daily.

Side-Effects:

Digitalis toxicity (Table 2). Virtually half of adverse reactions to toxicity are cardiac arrhythmias. Gastrointestinal disturbances account for one fourth, and CNS disturbances for one fourth of its toxic effects.

Nursing Implications:

Monitor cardiac rhythm for changes in rate and rhythm. Watch for signs of digitalis toxicity. Notify physician if any are noted.

TABLE 2. Digitalis Toxicity

Type of Toxicity	Toxic Effects
Cardiac	Premature ventricular contractions, especially ventricular bigeminy
	Ventricular tachycardia
	Ventricular fibrillation
	Nonparoxysmal A-V junctional tachycardia with or without block
	Atrial tachycardia with block or without; seen often in presence of hypokalemia caused by simultaneous use of thiazide diuretics
	Prolonged conduction through A-V node causing prolonged PR interval (1° A-V Block)
	Slowing of heart rate to bradycardia status; includes sinus bradycardia, 2° A-V Block: Mobitz I, and Complete Heart Block
Neurologic	Personality changes, mental depression
	Visual disturbances such as with colors green, brown, and yellow; blurred vision, dimmed vision, scotoma, photophobia, peripheral neuritis
	Cerebral irritation: headache, vertigo, increased irritability, convulsions
	Generalized muscular weakness
Gastro-intestinal	Anorexia
	Nausea and/or vomiting
	Diarrhea
Other	Allergic reactions such as skin rash
	Gynecomastica

DISOPYRAMIDE PHOSPHATE (Norpace)

Mechanism:

Lengthens conduction period
Decreases automaticity of myocardium
Vagolytic effect

Uses:

For treatment of supraventricular and ventricular arrhythmias. Better tolerated than quinidine.

Administration:

Maintenance dose of 150 to 200 mg every 6 hours. Patients weighing less than 50 kg or who have renal, hepatic, or cardiac impairment: 100 mg every 6 hours.

Side-Effects:

Most often reported: dry mouth, urinary hesitancy
Fatigue, dizziness, syncope, agitation, depression, muscle weakness
Hypotension, heart failure, heart block
Nausea, vomiting, anorexia, abdominal cramps, constipation
Urinary retention
Ventricular arrhythmias

Nursing Implications:

Monitor BP for hypotension.
Monitor ECG for occurrence of heart block and/or ventricular arrhythmias.
Check patient for early signs of side-effects and report to physician.

GLUCAGON

Mechanism:

Augmental impetus to cardiac contractility, even in presence of full digitalization or beta receptor blockage

Increases myocardial oxygen consumption by means of coronary bloodflow

Increases heart block

Decreases A-V conduction

Uses:

To reverse bradycardia caused by beta adrenergic receptor blocking agents. Produces less arrhythmias than Isuprel, but less effective in presence of heart failure.

Administration:

2.5 to 15 mg/hour IV in D5W.

Side-Effects:

Arrhythmias

Nausea and vomiting

Hypokalemia

Hyperglycemia at first; secondary hypoglycemia may result

Contraindications:

In presence of pheochromocytoma

In presence of uncontrolled arrhythmias

Starting dose reduced by one tenth in patients receiving monamine oxidase inhibitors

May have adverse effects in patients with hypovolemia

Enhances anticoagulant effects of warfarin

Nursing Implications:

Monitor for arrhythmias. Glucagon forms a precipitate in chloride solutions.

ISOPROTERENOL (Isuprel)

Mechanism:

Stimulates beta adrenergic receptors in heart, thus increasing heart rate and contractility.

Uses:

Improves pacemaker automaticity and allows for improved A-V conduction during heart block to increase ventricular rate.

In cardiogenic shock, increases cardiac output by counteracting vasoconstriction causing perfusion failure.

Administration:

0.5 to 4 mg/minute by IV solution.

Side-Effects:

Tachyarrhythmias, PVCs, V-tach, V-fib may result. When PVCs result from bradycardia, increasing heart rate with Isuprel may eliminate ectopic beats.

In presence of hypovolemia, hypotension occurs from vasodilating effect.

Headache, flushing, angina, nausea, dizziness, tremors, and diaphoresis may occur.

Nursing Implications:

Check BP every 2 to 3 minutes until stable.

Monitor intra-arterial pressure, if possible.

Titrate as ordered, using BP, CVP, cardiac rhythm, and urine output as guides to effectiveness.

Monitor CVP or PAWP.

Record urine output hourly.

IV infiltration may produce severe tissue damage; be especially on the alert for early infiltration.

LIDOCAINE, LIDOCAINE HCl (Xylocaine)

Mechanism:

izz   Increases electrical stimulation threshold of ventricles during diastole, and causes little, if any, effect on blood pressure or myocardial contractility. Does not slow conduction speed or depress cardiac excitability when used in normal doses.

Uses:

To suppress premature ventricular contractions or V-tach.

Effective against ventricular arrhythmias in presence of myocardial infarction, cardiac surgery or trauma, and during digitalis toxicity.

Administration:

IV loading dose: 50 to 100 mg IV push. For IV infusion, dilute 2 Gm Lidocaine in 500 cc D5W; administer at rate of 1 to 4 mg/minute. IV bolus of 50 to 100 mg may be repeated 1 to 4 times each hour as necessary, but rarely more than 4 times in an hour.

Side-Effects:

Usually dose-related and are first seen in patient's neurological status: restlessness, depression, sleepiness, dizziness, blurred vision, diplopia, sweating, confusion, dysphagia, and paresthesias. With large doses, hypotension, convulsion and coma may occur.

Nursing Implications:

Use cautiously, or not at all, in presence of slow heart rate, heart block, or intraventricular conduction delays.

Dosage is reduced in patients with hepatic disease and heart failure.

Use infusion pump for accurate infusion rate monitoring.

Do continuous ECG monitoring and watch for development of bradycardia, heart block, or breakthrough ventricular arrhythmias.

Monitor vital signs every 15 minutes until stable.

Observe patient for signs of toxicity; reduce dosage if signs are minimal. In severe reactions, stop infusion and notify physician immediately.

METARAMINOL BITARTRATE (Aramine)

Mechanism:

Similar in action to norepinephrine (Levophed):

- Causes increased systolic and diastolic pressures by its potent vasoconstricting action. Longer duration than Levophed. Reflex bradycardia may occur with pressure elevation. Atropine can be used to prevent bradycardia and increase cardiac output.
- Increases stroke volume.

Uses:

Primary drug of choice in treatment of hypotension.
Treatment of supraventricular tachycardia (SVT) by vagal stimulation

Administration:

May be given IM or IV for immediate blood pressure elevation:

- IM route—2 to 10 mg is usual
- IV route—dilute 15 to 100 mg Aramine in 500 D5W and titrate according to patient's response

Side-Effects:

Ventricular arrhythmias
Bradycardia
Tissue sloughing at site of IV if infiltration occurs

Nursing Implications:

Monitor BP constantly during IV administration.
Monitor heart rate and observe for arrhythmias.
Use extreme caution during IV infusion to prevent infiltration.

MEXILETINE (Mexitil)*

Mechanism:

Depresses myocardial automaticity
Prolongs activation time

Uses:

Treatment of ventricular arrhythmias, either acute or chronic. Its efficacy is similar to that of procainamide HCl (Pronestyl) and lidocaine (Xylocaine).

Administration:

Maintenance dose of 200 to 400 mg every 8 hours. (Available in 100- and 200-mg capsules.) Absorption is delayed and slightly incomplete in patients with myocardial infarction and those receiving narcotics or analgesics that retard gastric emptying.

Side-Effects:

Neurologic: tremor, diplopia, ataxia, confusion, nystagmus, and dizziness
Gastrointestinal: nausea, vomiting, dyspepsia
Cardiac: hypotension, bradycardia, or exacerbation of arrhythmia

Nursing Implications:

Check BP for hypotensive effects.
Monitor ECG for heart rate and increased arrhythmias.
Observe for early signs of side-effects and report to physician.

* Investigational in the United States

PHENYTOIN (Dilantin)

Mechanism:

Shortens action potential duration and refractory period of S-A and A-V nodes, and atrial and ventricular muscles, and depresses automaticity of atria. Conduction velocity is left unaffected, if not improved, if in abnormal depressed state.

Uses:

Most effective in treating digitalis-induced arrhythmias, especially ventricular arrhythmias. Also very effective in treating PVCs and nonparoxysmal A-V junctional tachycardia. Atrial tachycardia with block also responds quite effectively to Dilantin. A-fib flutter is unresponsive.

Administration:

1 Gm p.o. the first 24 hours in divided doses has been found effective as a loading dose, followed by 100 mg p.o. q.i.d. for 2 days, then maintenance dose of 300 mg p.o. in three divided doses.

IV Dilantin is administered slowly, 50 mg (over 2-minute intervals) to 100 mg (every 5 to 10 minutes) until arrhythmia subsides or toxic symptoms occur. Maximum dose is 1000 mg given slow IV push.

Side-Effects:

Hypotension may result if Dilantin is given too rapidly IV.

Cardiac arrest is a risk; use Dilantin cautiously in presence of sinus bradycardia, S-A or A-V block.

Phlebitis is another possible side-effect. Dilantin solution is extremely alkaline and needs to be well diluted if small veins are used with IV administration

When used concurrently with anticoagulants, the required dose of Dilantin may be found toxic because its metabolism is retarded by simultaneous therapy.

Nursing Implications:

Do not mix Dilantin with D5W, because crystallization will occur. Flush IV line with saline solution before and after administration.

Give p.o. drug with food or large glass of water in order to minimize gastric irritation.

Avoid IM route of administration because tissue irritation may result.

Dilantin is contraindicated in heart block, sinus bradycardia, and Stokes-Adams attacks. Use cautiously in patients with heart failure, hepatic or renal dysfunction, hypotension, myocardial insufficiency, and respiratory depression, and in elderly or debilitated patients.

Watch patients on Dilantin and other antiarrhythmic agents for signs of additive cardiac depression.

The difference between therapeutic and toxic blood levels of Dilantin is slight (blood levels greater than 20 mcg/ml may be toxic). If toxic symptoms occur, have blood drawn to determine level and hold drug.

Good oral hygiene must be maintained to minimize gingival hyperplasia.

Warn patient not to drink alcohol as he may lose control of previously stable antiarrhythmic effects.

POTASSIUM

Mechanism:

Major regulation of body potassium is provided by renal function. Certain disease states and drug therapy can alter normal blood serum level of potassium:

- Hypokalemia produces abnormalities of the myocardium with conduction defects, and increased automaticity, causing both supraventricular and ventricular arrhythmias, and sensitivity to digitalis.
- Low extracellular potassium level enhances ectopic pacemaker activity.

Uses:

To correct arrhythmias caused by digitalis intoxication, even though potassium serum levels may be normal.

To suppress ectopic activity not caused by digitalis excess, in the presence of those conditions producing hypokalemia (certain metabolic and kidney diseases, diarrhea, vomiting, diuretic therapy, and prolonged IV therapy using potassium-free fluids increasing extracellular fluid volume, reducing normal serum levels of potassium by volume alone).

Administration:

For severe potassium depletion for treatment of arrhythmias secondary to digitalis toxicity. KCl is given IV in doses of 30 to 60 mEq/500 to 1000 cc D5W at rate of approximately 0.5 mEq/minute initially with close observation of ensuing effects.

For routine prophylactic use for patients receiving both digitalis and diuretic therapy, potassium salts of 10 to 20 mEq 3 to 4 times daily.

For patients on salt restriction, KCl is available in 300- and 500-mg as well as 1-Gm tablets or liquid.

(*Note:* Effects of potassium administration are related to administration rate, the patient's pre-existing potassium level, and the ratio of intracellular and extracellular potassium concentrations.)

Side-Effects:

Rapid IV infusions of potassium can cause bradycardia, cellular pacemaker depression, and conduction slowing to extreme point of block.

Nausea, vomiting, diarrhea, and abdominal distress may occur.

Hyperkalemia may occur, with ECG manifestations of narrowed, peaked T waves and shortening of Q-T interval. Widening of QRS complex occurs with increasing toxicity, as PR interval lengthens and P wave diminishes in size or even disappears. ST segment may shift also. Changes of ECG usually appear when serum K^+ level reaches 7 to 8 mEq/liter.

Other clinical manifestations occur at 9 to 10 mEq/liter and may include muscle paralysis and death from cardiac arrest.

Nursing Implications:

Rapid IV administration may cause burning and/or pain at infusion site. (Some hospitals carry Neut, a solution that neutralizes the burning effect; one vial is added to IV solution along with KCl).

Contraindicated in presence of second-degree A-V block.

Contraindicated in patients with severe renal impairment with oliguria or azotemia, acute dehydration, acidosis, pre-existing hyperkalemia, and untreated Addison's disease.

Continuously monitor ECG and observe for occurrence of arrhythmias and/or block.

Note electrolyte levels daily, and even more frequently during initial IV potassium therapy.

PROCAINAMIDE HCl (Pronestyl)

Mechanism:

Refractory period is prolonged, more so in atria than in ventricles. Atrial and ventricular excitability is depressed. Pronestyl lengthens conduction time in cardiac muscle, Purkinje fibers, and A-V conduction tissues, and decreases automaticity of pacemaker cells.

Uses:

Primarily in treatment of PVCs and ventricular tachyarrhythmias when IV lidocaine has been used unsuccessfully. Used in low doses in combination with quinidine for treatment of atrial arrhythmias when quinidine alone is ineffective.

Administration:

IV loading dose: 50 to 100 mg diluted in D5W and given over a period of 30 minutes. For IV infusion, dilute 2 Gm procainamide HCl (Pronestyl) in 500 cc D5W; administer at rate of 2 to 4 mg/minute (usual dose, but can go as high as 6 mg/minute). IV Pronestyl has immediate effect.

Pronestyl usually is given IV or orally, but can be administered IM. After injection, peak levels are obtained in 15 minutes to 1 hour.

Oral loading dose is 500 mg to 1 Gm followed by 500 mg every 4 to 6 hours daily. In some patients with refractory arrhythmias, dosage may have to be as frequent as every 3 hours.

Side-Effects:

CNS: confusion, depression, hallucinations, convulsions.

CVS: bradycardia, severe hypotension, A-V block. Ventricular fibrillation may occur after IM administration.

GI: bitter taste, nausea, vomiting, anorexia, diarrhea.

A syndrome resembling lupus erythematosus can occur with oral therapy.

Other reactions include maculopapular rash, fever, and myalgia.

Nursing Implications:

Contraindicated in patients with second degree or complete heart block because it may cause asystole or advance the degree of block.

Use IV infusion pump to monitor infusion precisely.

During IV administration, continuously monitor ECG and watch for prolonged Q-T and Q-R intervals, heart block, or increased arrhythmias. Should any of these occur, obtain rhythm strip and notify physician.

Monitor ECG continuously until patient is stabilized on oral dosage.

Check BP and keep vasopressors close at hand to avert hypotensive crisis.

Do frequent blood-level checks if patient is on long-term therapy.

Watch patient closely for signs of side-effects and notify physician if they occur.

Patients with heart failure and renal or hepatic dysfunction can be treated with lesser dosages.

Stress to patient the importance of taking medication exactly as prescribed by the physician.

Restoration of normal sinus rhythm in patients with long-standing atrial fibrillation may result in thromboembolism because of dislodgment of thrombi from atrial wall. Thus, anticoagulation therapy is usually begun before restoration to normal sinus rhythm is attempted.

PROPRANOLOL HCl (Inderal)

Mechanism:

Decreases heart rate (automaticity of pacemakers is reduced). "Quinidine-like" antiarrhythmic effect prolongs A-V conduction and refractory period.

Uses:

Particularly effective for digitalis toxicity states when control of ectopic discharge is needed. Controls ventricular response to atrial tachyarrhythmias. In combination with quinidine sulfate, is an effective treatment for supraventricular tachyarrhythmias.

Administration:

0.5 to 1 mg per minute (or 2 minutes), up to 3 mg IV. Oral doses range from 10 to 80 mg three or four times daily.

Side-Effects:

Fatigue, lethargy, vivid dreams, hallucinations
Bradycardia, hypotension, heart failure
Nausea, vomiting, diarrhea
Hypoglycemia without tachycardia
Rash
Increased airway resistance, fever, impotence

Nursing Implications:

Should not be used in presence of heart failure, sinus bradycardia, or A-V block greater than first degree.

Withdraw drug slowly; quick withdrawal may precipitate myocardial infarction.

Double-check dose and route; IV doses are much smaller than p.o.

Monitor BP, ECG, heart rate, and rhythm frequently, especially during IV administration.

Check patient's lungs for rales, and heart for gallop rhythm or third or fourth heart sounds. Notify physician if any of these develop.

Monitor patient daily for weight gain or peripheral edema.

Check to be sure patient has no history of COPD prior to drug administration.

QUINIDINE, QUINIDINE SULFATE

Mechanism:

Decreases cardiac irritability, conduction speed, and myocardial contractility. Enhances A-V conduction by blocking vagal stimulation, causing increase in sinus node discharge rate.

Uses:

Treatment of most supraventricular arrhythmias not associated with heart block; especially successful with atrial fibrillation and atrial flutter.

Maintenance therapy after electrical shock conversion of atrial fibrillation or flutter.

Administration:

200 to 300 mg p.o. 3 or 4 times daily for PACs or PVCs.

400 to 600 mg every 2 to 3 hours for PAT until terminated.

With atrial fibrillation or flutter, 200 mg quinidine is given every 2 to 3 hours for 5 to 8 doses with daily increments until normal sinus rhythm is restored or toxic effects develop. Quinidine should only be given after digitalization in order to avoid increasing A-V conduction.

(*Note:* Maximum daily dose should not exceed 3 to 4 Gm in any therapeutic regimen.)

In presence of congestive heart failure, ventricular rate and failure should first be controlled by digitalis therapy.

Side-Effects:

CNS: Headache, dizziness, and vertigo, as well as confusion, fainting, pallor, cold sweat, blurred vision, and tinnitis may result from taking quinidine.

CVS: ECG changes may occur, such as PVCs, widening QRS complex, notched P waves, ST segment depression, widened Q-T interval, tachycardia, and possible ventricular fibrillation. Severe hypotension and aggravated congestive heart failure also result from taking quinidine.

GI: Nausea, vomiting, diarrhea, abdominal pain, and anorexia may occur.

Pulmonary side-effects include acute asthmatic attack and respiratory arrest.

Hematologic changes may occur, such as acute hemolytic anemia, thrombocytopenia, purpura, and agranulocytosis.

Dermatologic effects may include cutaneous flushing, intense pruritis, and subcutaneous hemorrhage of buccal mucosa.

Nursing Implications:

Use cautiously with patients previously digitalized, because quinidine may increase toxicity of digitalis. Monitor serum digoxin level.

Monitor ECG for changes in rate, rhythm, and complex configuration. Notify physician of any changes.

Dosage should be decreased in patients with congestive heart failure, or renal or hepatic dysfunction.

Gastrointestinal side-effects, especially diarrhea, are signs of quinidine toxicity; notify physician. Blood levels greater than 8 μg/ml are toxic.

Anticoagulation is often begun prior to restoration of normal sinus rhythm. Thromboembolism may result following long-standing atrial fibrillation or flutter due to dislodgment of thrombi from atrial wall.

If quinidine solution becomes brownish, discard.

Monitor for decreased quinidine effect if patient is concurrently on barbiturates, Dilantin, or rifampin.

Monitor for increased effect if patient is concurrently taking antacids, sodium bicarbonate or Diamox.

Do not use in combination with verapamil when patient has cardiomyopathy because it may result in severe hypotension.

Contraindicated when A-V conduction is severely impaired.

SODIUM BICARBONATE (NaHCO₃)

Mechanism:

Reverses metabolic acidosis.

Uses:

To correct metabolic acidosis resulting from ventricular fibrillation or cardiac arrest.

Administration:

Sodium bicarbonate is available in 44-mEq ampules or 500-ml IV bottles. Three to five ampules are usually given during cardiac arrest if patient is not immediately resuscitated. One ampule is given every 5 minutes until cardiopulmonary action is regained.

Side-Effects:

Overdosage produces metabolic alkalosis, and may also worsen pre-existing heart failure.

Nursing Implications:

Arterial blood gases must be closely observed during resuscitative procedures; administration of sodium bicarbonate is regulated by blood pH levels.

The underlying cause of acidosis should be identified if treatment with sodium bicarbonate is used. If the defect is perfusion failure, the condition may worsen with large amounts of sodium-based fluid.

Thoroughly flush IV line before and after administration, because other drugs are incompatible with sodium bicarbonate. (If you can, establish two IV lines, to decrease possibility of drug incompatibility as well as for speed of giving drugs in an emergency situation.)

Watch for signs of heart failure.

TOCAINIDE* (Tonocard)

Mechanism:

Reduces automaticity of pacemaker cells and prolongs activation time.

Uses:

Chronic ventricular ectopy and arrhythmias.

Administration:

Available in 400-mg capsules. Give 400 to 800 mg every 8 hours orally. (Also available in IV form.)

Side-Effects:

Cardiovascular effects include hypotension, brady-cardia, palpitations, chest pain, conduction disturbances, left ventricular heart failure, and increased ventricular arrhythmias.

Other effects are as follows:

Gastrointestinal upsets

Neurological disturbances including

       Headache

       Hot flashes

       Tremors

       Altered hearing

       Diaphoresis

       Parasthesia

Nursing Implications

Monitor cardiac rhythm.

Observe for signs of toxicity, especially neurologic changes.

---

* A major amine analog of lidocaine.

VERAPAMIL (Isoptin, Calan)

Mechanism:

Blocks calcium from crossing cell membrane
Reduces extent of myocardial ischemia
Depresses S-A node discharge rate
Prolongs A-V node conduction
Depresses myocardial contractility

Uses:

Effective in treating paroxysmal supraventricular tachycardias.

Slows ventricular response to A-fib flutter.

Prophylactic treatment for recurrent PAT and supraventricular tachycardias.

Also used for treating angina pectoris by means of coronary vasodilation.

Administration:

5 to 10 mg IV push over 1 minute with ECG and BP monitoring. Repeat dose in 30 minutes if there is no response. Maintenance infusion of 0.005 mg/kg/minute may follow IV bolus.

Side-Effects:

Dizziness, headache, fatigue
Transient hypotension, heart failure; more rarely, bradycardia, A-V block, ventricular asystole, peripheral edema
Constipation, nausea
Elevated liver enzymes

Nursing Implications:

Should be avoided in presence of sick sinus syndrome, A-V conduction problems, and severe heart failure.

Use cautiously with beta blockers.

IV doses should be administered over at least 3 minutes in older patients to minimize adverse effects.

Notify physician if swelling of hands and feet occurs, or shortness of breath—all signs of heart failure.

Monitor cardiac rhythm and watch for A-V block or bradycardia.

Closely check BP, noting hypotensive changes.

Appendix II:

The Twelve-Lead

Electrocardiogram

The standard electrocardiogram (ECG) is composed of twelve leads: six limb (bipolar) leads and six chest (unipolar) leads. To obtain limb leads, electrodes are placed on the right and left arms and left leg, forming Einthoven's triangle (Fig. 14). An electrode sensor is placed on the right leg to stabilize the tracing. The limb leads form the frontal plane of the chest.

Lead I is horizontal: right arm equals negative, left arm equals positive

Lead II is vertical: right arm equals negative, left leg equals positive

Lead III is vertical: left leg equals positive, left arm equals negative

AVR (Augmented Voltage Right Arm): right arm equals positive and all other sensors are channeled into a common ground

AVL (Augmented Voltage Left Arm): left arm equals positive

AVF (Augmented Voltage Left Foot): left foot equals positive

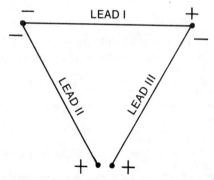

Fig. 14. Einthoven's triangle.

In all chest leads, the electrode sensor placed on the chest is positive and covers the heart in its anatomical position within the chest. (The indifferent electrode consists of left arm, right arm, and left leg).

Figure 15 shows correct positioning of chest leads.

Steps in Running ECG

1. **Standardize:** make sure stylus rises exactly 10 small squares (1 cm) before it returns to baseline.
2. Do limb leads first and mark as follows:
   Lead I: one short line   -
   Lead II: two short lines   --

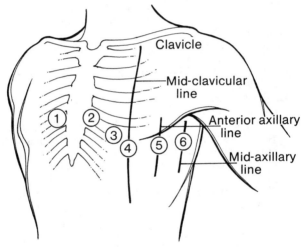

Fig. 15. Positioning of chest leads.

V_1: fourth intercostal space to right of sternum, usually over right atrium

V_2: fourth intercostal space to left of sternum, usually over right ventricle

V_3: halfway between V_2 & V_4, usually over ventricular septal area.

V_4: fifth intercostal space in midclavicular line, usually over septum of left ventricle.

V_5: fifth intercostal space in anterior axillary line, usually over left ventricle.

V_6: fifth intercostal space in midaxillary line, usually over left ventricle.

Lead III: three short lines - - -
AVR: four short lines   - - - -
AVL: five short lines   - - - - -
AVF: six short lines   - - - - - -

3. Chest leads are preceded by a long dash, then the number of short lines representing the number of the chest lead.

V_1: — -
V_2: — - -
V_3: — - - -
V_4: — - - - -
V_5: — - - - - -
V_6: — - - - - - -

4. In Lead I and Lead V_6, depress standard button between complexes once on each lead to make certain machine is still correctly standardized.
5. Return knob to "on" position between each lead.
6. Run approximately 6 inches of each lead.
7. Have patient relax as much as possible during the ECG. If all other attempts to help patient relax fail, have him put his hands under his buttocks.

Some of the newer ECG machines have six chest lead electrodes which allow for all leads to be positioned at the same time. This means an ECG may be taken more rapidly, making it more convenient for the nurse and easier on the patient.

Appendix III:

Self-Evaluation

Choose the best answer to the following questions, and check yourself with the answers provided at the end of this section.

1. The most common complication of acute myocardial infarction is
   A. Arrhythmias.
   B. Some degree of congestive heart failure.
   C. Ventricular rupture.
   D. Recurrent and persistent pain.

2. Number, in order, the actions that should be taken in the event a patient suddenly develops ventricular fibrillation while you are at the bedside.
   _____ Initiate CPR and summon help.
   _____ Administer a lidocaine bolus.
   _____ Administer sodium bicarbonate.
   _____ Defibrillate as soon as possible.

3. Electromechanical dissociation is best treated by
   A. Adrenalin, sodium bicarbonate, and calcium.
   B. Immediate defibrillation.
   C. Isuprel, calcium, and sodium bicarbonate.
   D. Atropine, Isuprel, and lidocaine.

4. Digitalis toxicity can cause
   A. Rhythm disturbances.
   B. Nausea and vomiting.
   C. Hypokalemia.
   D. Decreased renal function.
   E. All of the above.
   F. None of the above.

5. A PVC on the T wave of the preceding beat
   A. Can be ignored if less common than 6 per minute.
   B. Can be ignored if less common than 3 per minute.
   C. Needs to be treated.
   D. Will reset the atrial rhythm.
   E. Requires no treatment.

6. The sinus node
   A. Normally discharges at a rate of 60 to 100.
   B. Is located in the left atrium.
   C. Is discharged by an impulse arising in the A-V node.
   D. Is depolarized during the contraction of the right ventricle.

7. The atrial rate in atrial fibrillation is
   A. 100 to 250
   B. 250 to 350
   C. 200 to 250
   D. 350 to infinity

8. A prolonged PR interval (greater than 0.20 second) indicates
   A. Malfunction of the sinus node.
   B. Delayed conduction of the A-V node.
   C. Mobitz II.
   D. Third degree A-V block.

9. Second degree A-V block, Mobitz Type I (Wenckebach) is characterized by
   A. Progressive shortening of the PR interval.
   B. A broad QRS complex.
   C. Progressive lengthening of PR interval with a short PR interval in the cycle following the nonconducted P wave.
   D. Progressive lengthening in the P-P interval.

10. A PAC (premature atrial contraction)
    A. Is characterized by a normal P wave.
    B. Originates in the S-A node.
    C. Originates in the atria.
    D. Should be treated with Lidocaine.

11. The A-V junction depolarizes at a rate of
    A. 20 to 40 times per minute.
    B. 40 to 60 times per minute.
    C. 60 to 100 times per minute.
    D. It does not have the property of automaticity.

12. The QRS complex begins when the impulse reaches the
    A. Bundle of His.
    B. A–V node.
    C. Ventricular muscle.
    D. Left bundle branch.

13. A PVC
   A. Can arise from either ventricle.
   B. Is always of the same configuration in the same patient.
   C. Must be treated immediately.
   D. Is always followed by a compensatory pause.

14. Ventricular tachycardia is almost always regular.
   A. True
   B. False

15. Complete heart block can seriously decrease cardiac output and cause shock.
   A. True
   B. False

16. Lidocaine can increase conduction rate across the A-V node.
   A. True
   B. False

17. In PAT (paroxysmal atrial tachycardia), the ventricular rate is usually irregular.
   A. True
   B. False

18. Ventricular fibrillation is first treated with lidocaine, then cardioversion.
   A. True
   B. False

19. Lidocaine is used to treat PVCs in third degree A-V block.
   A. True
   B. False

20. An inverted P wave of less than 0.12 second preceding a normal QRS in a premature beat is indicative of a premature junctional ectopic.
   A. True
   B. False

For the following rhythm strips, you will need your calipers. After making the appropriate measurements, write your complete diagnosis (interpretation). Spaces are provided for your answers.

21.

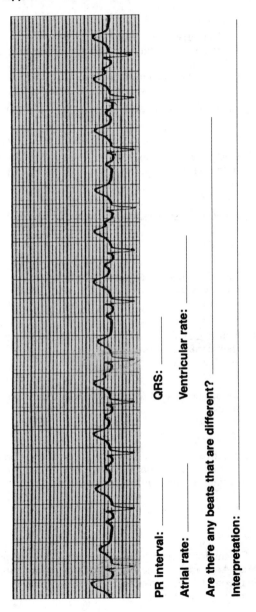

PR interval: _____   QRS: _____

Atrial rate: _____   Ventricular rate: _____

Are there any beats that are different? _____

Interpretation: _____

22.

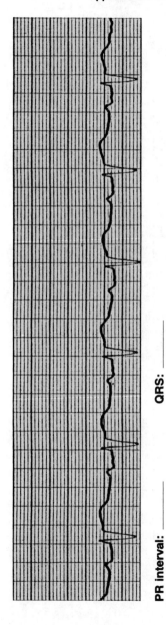

PR interval: _____   QRS: _____

Atrial rate: _____   Ventricular rate: _____

Are there any beats that are different? _____

Interpretation: _____

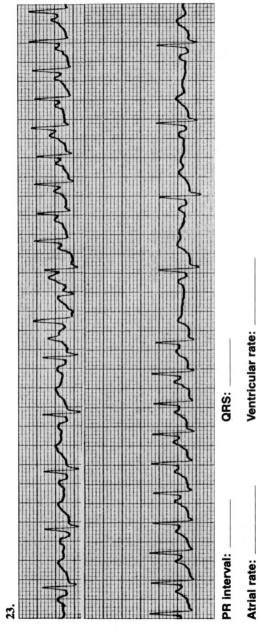

23.

PR interval: _____   QRS: _____

Atrial rate: _____   Ventricular rate: _____

Are there any beats that are different? _____

Interpretation: _____

150

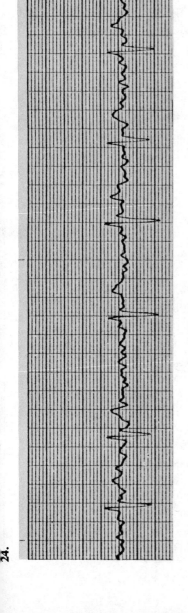

24.

PR interval: _____   **QRS:** _____

Atrial rate: _____   **Ventricular rate:** _____

Are there any beats that are different? _____

Interpretation: _____

25.

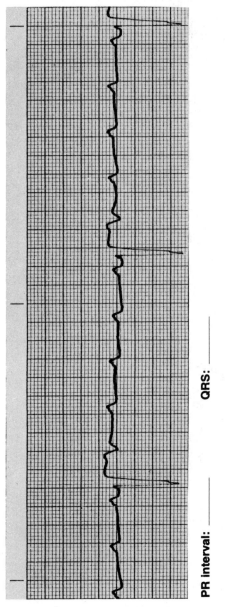

PR interval: _____   QRS: _____

Atrial rate: _____   Ventricular rate: _____

Are there any beats that are different? _____

Interpretation: _____

26.

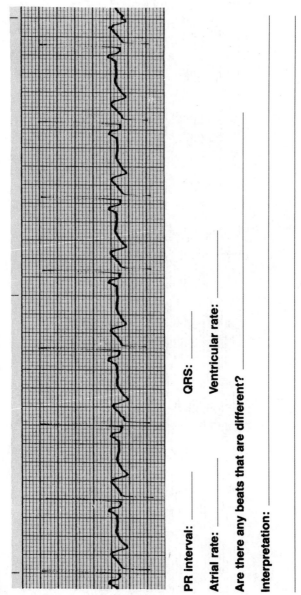

PR interval: _____   QRS: _____

Atrial rate: _____   Ventricular rate: _____

Are there any beats that are different? _____

Interpretation: _____

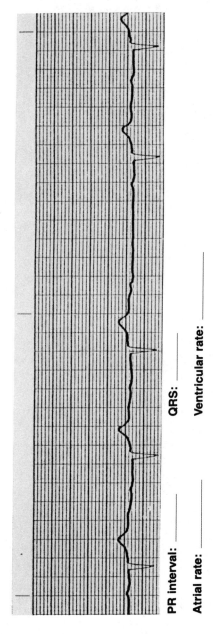

PR interval: _____   **QRS:** _____

Atrial rate: _____   **Ventricular rate:** _____

Are there any beats that are different? _____

Interpretation: _____

_____

27.

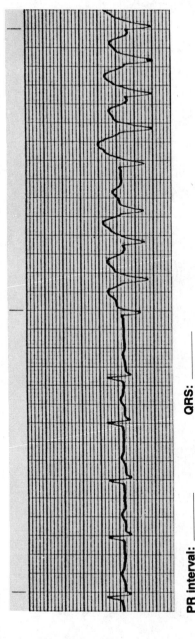

PR interval: _____ QRS: _____

Atrial rate: _____ Ventricular rate: _____

Are there any beats that are different? _____

Interpretation: _____

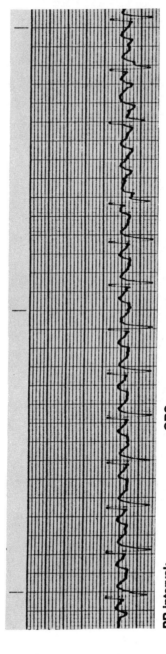

29.

PR interval: _____   QRS: _____

Atrial rate: _____   Ventricular rate: _____

Are there any beats that are different? _____

Interpretation: _____

_____

30.

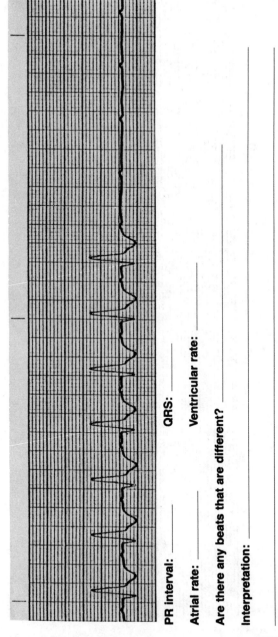

PR interval: —————   QRS: —————

Atrial rate: —————   Ventricular rate: —————

Are there any beats that are different? —————

Interpretation: —————

157

31.

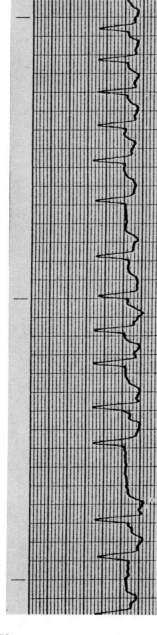

PR interval: _____ QRS: _____

Atrial rate: _____ Ventricular rate: _____

Are there any beats that are different? _____

Interpretation: _____

32.

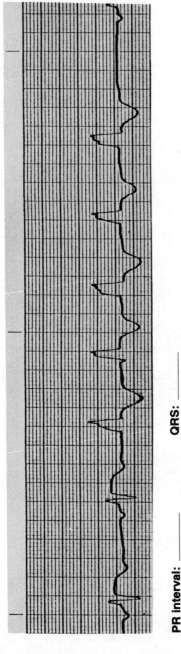

PR interval: _____   QRS: _____

Atrial rate: _____   Ventricular rate: _____

Are there any beats that are different? _____

Interpretation: _____

159

33.

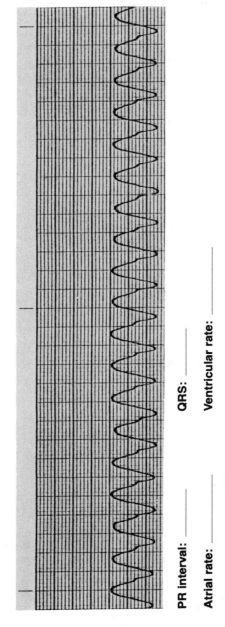

PR interval: _____   QRS: _____

Atrial rate: _____   Ventricular rate: _____

Are there any beats that are different? _____

Interpretation: _____

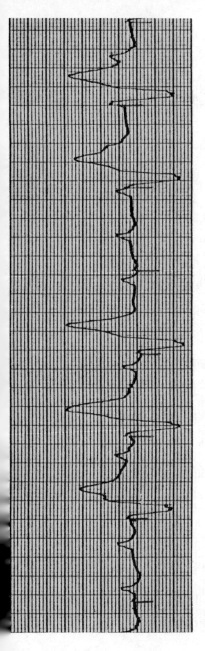

PR interval: ———

QRS: ——— Ventricular rate: ———

Atrial rate: ———

Are there any beats that are different? ———

Interpretation: ———

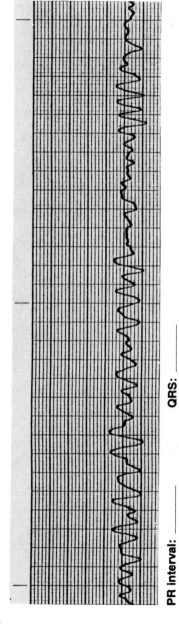

35.

PR interval: _____   QRS: _____

Atrial rate: _____   Ventricular rate: _____

Are there any beats that are different? _____

Interpretation: _____
_____

Answers to Self-Evaluation Questions

1. A—Arrhythmias. Some cardiologists prefer to place patient on prophylactic lidocaine drip until critical period is over.

2. 1 —Initiate CPR and summon help.
   3 —Administer a lidocaine bolus.
   4 —Administer sodium bicarbonate.
   2 —Defibrillate *as soon as possible.*

3. A—Adrenalin, sodium bicarbonate, and calcium

4. E—All of the above

5. C—This is R-on-T phenomenon (PVC falling in vulnerable period) and can easily precipitate ventricular tachycardia.

6. A—Normal discharge rate of sinus node is 60 to 100 per minute.

7. D—350 to infinity. At times, undulations in baseline are barely visible due to rapidity of atrial discharge.

8. B—Delayed conduction of the A-V node.

9. C—Wenckebach is characterized by progressive lengthening of PR interval until a nonconducted P wave occurs; then the cycle begins again.

10. C—A PAC is a premature ectopic beat originating in atria.

11. B—The depolarization rate of the A-V junction is 40 to 60 times per minute.

12. C—Ventricular muscle

13. A—PVCs can arise from either ventricle. (Remember, interpolated PVCs have no compensatory pause.)

14. A (True)—May rarely be irregular if PVCs arise from several different foci.

15. A (True)—Atria and ventricles beat independently with slow ventricular rate leading to decreased cardiac output.

16. A (True)—Lidocaine increases electrical stimulation threshold of ventricles during diastole and does not slow conduction speed.

17. B (False)—Ventricular rate is regular.

18. B (False)—Initiate CPR and defibrillate as soon as possible.

19. B (False)—Lidocaine could completely knock out ventricular activity.

20. A (True)—Inverted P wave of less than 0.12 second arises from A-V junctional tissue.

21. Sinus tachycardia with frequent PACs
PR: .16
QRS: .08
Atrial rate: 107
Ventricular rate: 107

22. Normal sinus rhythm with 1° A-V block and bundle branch block
PR: .28
QRS: .12
Atrial rate: 63
Ventricular rate: 63

23. (1) Normal sinus rhythm ⟶ (2) PAC ⟶ (3) parox-ysmal atrial tachycardia ⟶ (4) normal sinus rhythm
PR: (1) & (4) .14
QRS: (1) & (4) .08
Atrial rate: (1) & (4) 100, 79
Ventricular rate: (1) 100   (3) 188   (4) 79

24. Coarse atrial fibrillation
PR: —
QRS: .11
Atrial rate: rapid, irregular
Ventricular rate: approximately 60, irregular

25. 2° A-V block, Mobitz Type II and bundle branch block
PR: —
QRS: .12
Atrial rate: 120
Ventricular rate: 25

26. Normal sinus rhythm
PR: .16
QRS: .06
Atrial rate: 75
Ventricular rate: 75

27. 2° A-V block, Mobitz Type I (Wenckebach)
PR: .28 to .42
QRS: .08
Atrial rate: irregular
Ventricular rate: 50 (making it bradycardia)

28. (1) Atrial fibrillation ⟶ (2) irregular ventricular
tachycardia ⟶ (3) ventricular tachycardia (regular)
PR: —
QRS: (1) .08   (2) .16   (3) .16
Atrial rate: (1) rapid, irregular
Ventricular rate: (1) 100   (3) 168

29. Atrial flutter with 2 : 1 and 4 : 1 ventricular response
PR: —
QRS: .10
Atrial rate: 250
Ventricular rate: approximately 120

30. (1) Sinus tachycardia with bundle branch block ⟶
(2) ventricular asystole
PR: (1) .16   (2) —
QRS: (1) .14   (2) —
Atrial rate: (1) & (2) 104
Ventricular rate: (1) 104   (2) none

31. Atrial fibrillation with rapid ventricular response
PR: —
QRS: .08 to .10
Atrial rate: rapid, irregular
Ventricular rate: 140

32. (1) Sinus bradycardia ⟶ (2) accelerated idioventric-
ular rhythm (slow V-tach) ⟶ (3) sinus rhythm
PR: (1) .16   (2) none
QRS: (1) .10   (2) .16
Atrial rate: (1) 56   (2) none
Ventricular rate: (1) 56   (2) 79

33. Ventricular tachycardia
PR: —
QRS: .16
Atrial rate: none
Ventricular rate: 188 regular

34. Pacemaker firing at rate of 70 with two episodes of noncapture. Possible underlying rhythm of 2° or 3° A-V block.
PR: —
QRS: .18
Atrial rate: 125
Ventricular rate: 70

35. Coarse ventricular fibrillation
PR: —
QRS: different widths
Atrial rate: none
Ventricular rate: rapid, irregular at approximately 350 to 400

Glossary

Aberrancy: deviation of impulse conduction from normal pathway, reflected by altered ECG configuration.

Arrest: cessation of heart's contractile activity; can refer to either atrial or ventricular arrest.

Arrhythmia: abnormalities of impulse formation and conduction. More specifically, refers to variation from normal rate and sequences of cardiac activity.

Artifact: extraneous mechanical or electrical interference on ECG or cardiac monitor not caused by heart's electrical activity.

Asynchronous Electronic Pacemaker: unit that continuously delivers electrical impulses to ventricular myocardium.

Asystole: absence of cardiac contractions. Refers either to entire heart or a pair of chambers, *e.g.*, ventricular asystole.

Atrial Arrest: cessation of atrial contractions.

Atrial Fibrillation: uncoordinated atrial activity. Represented on ECG by continuous, irregular deviations from baseline.

Atrial Flutter: distinct and rapid atrial depolarization from an atrial pacemaker (generally at rate of 300).

Atrial Tachycardia: rapid, repetitive contractions arising from ectopic atrial focus.

Atrioventricular (A-V) Block: conduction defect in A-V node or major conduction bundles. Varying degrees of block: 1° A-V block = excessive slowing (greater than 0.20 second) of conduction time of sinus impulses as they pass through A-V conduction pathway; 2° A-V block = intermittent failure of impulses from sinus node to completely transverse A-V conduction pathway; 3° A-V block = complete failure of all impulses to penetrate A-V conduction pathway.

Atrioventricular (A-V) Dissociation: atria and ventricles beat independently, each under control of separate pacemakers.

Atrioventricular (A-V) Node: specialized conducting fibers through which impulses pass between atria and ventricles. Located at base of atrial septum above ventricular septum.

Atrium: upper contractile chamber of heart. Right atrium receives oxygen-poor venous blood from superior and inferior vena cava ejecting it into right ventricle. Left atrium receives oxygenated blood from pulmonary veins and ejects it into left ventricle.

Beat: one complete mechanical and electrical cardiac cycle.

Bigeminy: generally refers to sinus beats alternating with ectopic beats. Paired cardiac contractions in recurring pattern each from a separate pacemaker. Rhythm is designated by ectopic pacemaker, *e.g.,* atrial, nodal, or ventricular bigeminy.

Block: delay or obstruction of impulse conduction.

Bradycardia: slowing of cardiac rate below defined limits. Sinus bradycardia: less than 60 per minute. Nodal bradycardia: less than 40 per minute. Ventricular bradycardia: less than 20 per minute.

Bundle: tract of impulse conducting fibers.

Bundle of His: common bundle. Fibers leading from A-V node to branches in ventricles. Right bundle branch: fibers from bundle of His distributed to endocardial surface of right ventricle. Left bundle branch: fibers from bundle of His distributed to endocardial surface of left ventricle; fibers divide into an anterior and a posterior branch before reaching endocardial surface.

Cadence: established rhythm of cardiac impulse formation.

Capture: depolarization of a cardiac chamber by a stimulus. Most commonly refers to activation of chamber by electronic pacemaker; current stimulates heart muscle and heartbeat results from impulse.

Cardiac Arrest: general term describing sudden collapse from ineffective cardiac contractions; includes ventricular arrest or fibrillation.

Compensatory Pause: delay in ventricular systole following a premature contraction occurring in sinus rhythm. Eliminates a sinus beat but does not interfere with sinus cadence. Interval between R waves of normal sinus beat preceding and following premature beat is double that of normal R-R interval.

Complete A-V Block: absence of impulse conduction between atria and ventricles. (also, *complete heart block, 3° A-V block*).

Conduction: transmission of depolarizing impulse through cardiac tissue.

Contraction: shortening of cardiac muscle fibers causing decrease in volume of chamber.

Coupling: pairing of beats, two in a row; generally refers to ectopic beats.

Deflection: deviation of ECG line from baseline.

Demand Electronic Pacemaker: device that is programmed to initiate ventricular conduction when normal cardiac activation is absent.

Depolarization: activation of automatic, conductile, and contractile tissue from polarized (resting) state.

Diastole: relaxation and dilation of cardiac chambers; is rhythmic.

Dissociation: independent beating of atria and ventricles.

Ectopic: impulse originating outside sinus node.

Electrocardiogram (ECG): recording of heart's electrical activity by series of deflections which reflect components of cardiac cycle.

Electrocardiograph: instrument for recording heart's electrical activity.

Electrode: conducting terminal which completes electrical circuit between transmitting and receiving device. Used when referring to electrocardiographs, cardiac monitors, and pacemakers.

Endocardium: heart's inner layer; composed of connective tissue.

Epicardium: heart's outer layer; composed of connective tissue.

Escape Beat: ectopic contraction, originating outside sinus node, in which ectopic pacemaker is released by depression of formation of sinus impulses.

Excitability: capacity to respond to stimulation.

Excitation: any stimulating effect on heart that accelerates rate of impulse formation or velocity of conduction.

Exit Block: failure of impulse conduction from its origin to adjacent tissue (*e.g.*, sinoatrial block).

Extrasystole: ectopic premature beat (also premature contraction).

Fasicle: same as *bundle.*

Fibrillation: continuous, disorganized electrical and contractile activity of heart's chambers.

Fixed-Rate Electronic Pacemaker: unit that continuously delivers electrical impulses to ventricular myocardium (same as asynchronous pacemaker).

Flutter: rapid impulse formation with coordinated activity of paired cardiac chambers (as in atrial flutter).

Focus: site of cardiac tissue with capability of impulse formation.

Fusion Beat: cardiac contraction produced by two merging depolarizing waves from impulses originating from separate foci.

Idio-: prefix used when referring to ectopic rhythms; implies self-generated impulse formation (*e.g.,* idionodal, idioventricular).

Infarction: area of tissue necrosis due to cessation of blood supply.

Inhibited Response: used when referring to pacemaker programming: pacemaker fires only in absence of cardiac activity. Pacemaker resets self, *i.e.,* will not fire when electrical potentials are sensed.

Interpolated: used when referring to ectopic premature contractions that do not prevent formation of subsequent sinus beat. Appears as extra beat between two normal uninterrupted beats.

Junctional: tissue adjacent to A-V node and bundle of His with potential for automaticity. Origin of nodal (junctional) rhythm.

Junctional Premature Contraction: premature contraction originating in A-V junctional tissue (also called *nodal premature contraction*).

Leads: (1) electrical conductors through which body's electrical activity is sent to a recording device. (2) electrical conducting wire which carries electrical current from pacemaker's pulse generator to heart.

Mobitz Phenomenon: refers to Type II form of 2° A-V block; consists of intermittent blocked sinus beats (P waves without subsequent QRS complexes) with constant PR intervals of conducted beats.

Multifocal: used when referring to ectopic beats originating from two or more sites of impulse formation.

Multiform: same as *multifocal*.

Myocardium: muscle mass of heart.

Nodal Premature Contraction: premature contraction originating in A-V junctional tissue (also called *junctional premature contraction*).

Nodal Rhythm: series of contractions originating in A-V junctional tissue at rate of 40 to 60 per minute (also referred to as *junctional rhythm*).

Nodal Tachycardia: series of contractions originating in A-V junctional tissue at rate greater than 60 per minute.

P Wave: atrial depolarization as represented on ECG.

P-P Interval: duration of one complete cardiac cycle.

Pacemaker: (1) cell or cells that spontaneously depolarize forming impulses which initiate cardiac contraction. (2) electronic pulse generator.

Parasystole: regular contractions initiated by ectopic pacemaker unrelated to dominant rhythm.

Paroxysmal: sudden onset and cessation of recurring episodes of cardiac arrhythmias.

PR Interval: portion of ECG cycle measured from beginning of P wave to beginning of QRS complex.

Pulse Interval: period of time between two paced beats.

Pulse Width: period of time during which pacemaker stimulus is delivered to heart.

Purkinje Fibers: conductile fibers in ventricles' subendocardial tissues.

Q Wave: first negative ECG deflection of ventricular depolarization complex.

R Wave: first positive deflection on ECG of ventricular depolarization complex.

R-R Interval: distance between two consecutive R waves; represents duration of one cardiac cycle.

Refractory Period: repolarization interval during which there is decreased degree of excitability for subsequent depolarizing stimuli.

Repolarization: restoration to normal resting electrical polarity following depolarization.

Retrograde: impulse conduction in reverse or backward direction. Generally refers to A-V node.

S Wave: negative deflection on ECG which occurs after R wave of ventricular depolarization complex.

Septum: fibrous and muscular partition which separates right and left cardiac chambers.

Sick Sinus Syndrome: abnormal variability of sinus node impulse formation rate, having periods of rapid and slow pacemaker activity (also, *sinus syndrome, tachybradycardia syndrome*).

Sinoatrial Block: form of exit block whereby impulses formed in sinus node fail to be conducted.

Sinus Node: normal pacemaker of the heart. Group of specialized myocardial cells with automatic activity located in right atrial tissue.

Sinus Pause: momentary cessation of sinus node's automaticity.

Sinus Rhythm: natural cardiac rhythm originating from sinus node pacemaker; normal rate is 60 to 100 per minute.

Supraventricular: site above or proximal to ventricles (*e.g.*, S-A node, atria, A-V node).

Synchronous Electronic Pacemaker: device that artificially stimulates myocardium to ventricular activation following atrial contraction.

Systole: rhythmic contractions of cardiac chambers.

T Wave: ventricular repolarization as represented on ECG.

Tachyarrhythmia: rapid heart beat from any focus of automaticity.

Tachycardia: acceleration of cardiac rate above defined limits. Sinus tachycardia: greater than 100 per minute. Nodal tachycardia: greater than 60 per minute. Ventricular tachycardia: (a) accelerated idioventricular rhythm from 50 to 100; (b) ventricular tachycardia, greater than 100.

Threshold: amount of electrical energy required to stimulate response in automatic, conductile, and contractile tissue.

Trigeminy: recurring pattern of three beats, in which third beat is a premature contraction.

Triggered Response: pacemaker fires impulse every time it senses cardiac electrical potential.

Unifocal: ectopic beats originating from single site (also, *uniformed*).

Ventricle: contractile chamber of heart. Right ventricle: receives venous blood from right atrium and ejects it into pulmonary artery. Left ventricle: receives arterial blood from left atrium and ejects it into aorta. The left ventricle is the major muscular chamber of the heart.

Ventricular Arrest: cessation of ventricular contractions (also called *ventricular standstill*).

Ventricular Bradycardia: slowing of idioventricular rate to less than 20 per minute.

Ventricular Fibrillation: continuous, uncoordinated twitching of ventricles resulting in cessation of circulatory flow; caused by multifocal and asynchronous contractions of ventricles.

Ventricular Flutter: very rapid ventricular rhythm; on ECG, QRS complexes merge into T waves without detectable separation.

Ventricular-Inhibited Electronic Pacemaker: ventricular conduction is initiated by pacemaker when normal activation is absent.

Ventricular Premature Contraction: ventricular beat occurring early in normal cardiac cycle; characterized by prolonged and distorted QRS and T wave formation.

Ventricular Rhythm: sustained impulse formation from a ventricular focus; rate of 20 to 40 per minute.

Ventricular Tachycardia: rhythm caused by accelerated firing of automatic focus (or foci) within ventricles. Rate greater than 100 per minute.

Vulnerable Period: period during repolarization in which tissue is supersensitive to stimulation, and subthreshold stimuli may produce electrical instability. Stimuli during this interval tend to induce sustained rhythms of excitation, *e.g.,* tachycardia, fibrillation, flutter.

Wandering Pacemaker: impulse formation shifts from various sites within sinus node, atria, and A-V junctional tissue, causing variation in rhythmicity, P wave contour, and PR intervals.

Watt-Second: unit of electrical energy. Expresses amount of current exerted over time. (One watt-second = one joule.)

Wenckebach Phenomenon: form of 2° A-V block whereby PR intervals progressively lengthen in consecutive cardiac cycles until interrupted by block sinus beat. (Also called *2° A-V block, Mobitz Type I*).

Bibliography

American Heart Association: The American Heart Association Heartbook: A Guide to Prevention and Treatment of Cardiovascular Diseases, Chaps 6, 8, 12, 21. New York, EP Dutton, 1980

Andreoli KG, Fowkes VH, Zipes DP, Wallace AG: Comprehensive Cardiac Care: A Text for Nurses, Physicians and Other Health Practitioners, 4th ed, pp 128–233, 258–260, 335–373. St Louis, CV Mosby, 1979

Angel JE (pub): Physician's Desk Reference, 37th ed. Oradell, New Jersey, Medical Economics Company, 1983

Bates B: A Guide to Physical Examination, 3rd ed, pp 155–166. Philadelphia, JB Lippincott, 1983

Cantwell R, Hollis R, Rogers MP: Think fast: What do you know about cardiac drugs for a code? Nursing 82 (Oct):34–40, 1982

Combatting Cardiovascular Diseases Skillfully, pp 175–178. Springhouse, Pennsylvania, Nursing 82 Books, Intermed Communications, 1982

Ellis PD, Billings DM: Cardiopulmonary Resuscitation: Procedures for Basic and Advanced Life Support, pp 153–156. St Louis, CV Mosby, 1980

Giving Cardiovascular Drugs Safely, pp 71–84, 135–146. Springhouse, Pennsylvania, Nursing 82 Books, Intermed Communications, 1982

Goldberger E: Treatment of Cardiac Emergencies, 3rd ed, pp 59–138, 307–400. St Louis, CV Mosby, 1982

Kroncke GM, Gray J, Boake WC, Brown L: What to do when your patient's pacemaker stops working. Nursing 81 (Oct):73–78, 1981

Lasche PA: Permanent cardiac pacing: Technology and follow-up. Focus on Critical Care 10(5):28–36, 1983

Marriott HJL: Practical Electrocardiography, 6th ed, pp 99–167. Baltimore, Williams & Wilkins, 1977

Marriott HJL, Boudreau Conover MH: Advanced Concepts in Arrhythmias. St Louis, CV Mosby, 1983

Millar S, Sampson LK, Soukup SM, Weinberg SL (eds): Methods in Critical Care: The AACN Manual by the American Association of Critical-Care Nurses, pp1–29, 37–41. Philadelphia, WB Saunders, 1980

Nursing 84 Drug Handbook, pp 124–141, 170–171. Springhouse, Pennsylvania, Nursing 84 Books, Intermed Communications, 1984

Parsonnet V, Furman S, Smyth NPD: A revised code for pacemaker identification. Pacemaker study group. Circulation 64:60A–62A, 1981

Parsonnet V, Manhardt M: Permanent pacing of the heart: 1952–1976. Am J Cardiol 39:250–256, 1977

Phillips RE, Feeney MK: The Cardiac Rhythms: A Systematic Approach to Interpretation, 2nd ed, pp 55–325. Philadelphia, WB Saunders, 1980

Schamroth L: An Introduction to Electrocardiography, 6th ed, pp 147–278. St Louis, Blackwell Mosby Book Distributors, 1982

Slusarczyk SM, Hicks FD: Helping your patient to live with a permanent pacemaker. Nursing 83 (Apr):58–63, 1983

Sweetwood HM: Clinical Electrocardiography for Nurses, Chaps 1–5, 9. Rockville, Maryland, Aspen Systems, 1983

Van Meter M, Lavine PG: Reading EKGs Correctly, pp 29–84, 144–153. Horsham, Pennsylvania, Nursing 79 Books, Intermed Communications, 1979

Index

Page numbers followed by *f* indicate illustrations; *t* following a page number indicates tabular material.